Emotional Eating

Find Out Negative Emotions behind Your Hunger and Build a Healthy

(Step-by-step Guide to End Your Battle with Food and Satisfy Your Soul)

Richard Peters

Published By **Jordan Levy**

Richard Peters

Emotional Eating: Find Out Negative Emotions behind Your Hunger and Build a Healthy (Step-by-step Guide to End Your Battle with Food and Satisfy Your Soul)

ISBN   978-1-998769-06-3

Legal & Disclaimer

TABLE OF CONTENTS

Introduction

Do you feel like a prisoner to your emotions? When they come on fast and strong, how do you respond? Do you turn to food as your rescue? If so, you are most likely an emotional eater. While everyone "eats their feelings" on occasion, emotional eaters depend on food for comfort. This can have unwanted mental and physical consequences. How do you break free from these patterns?

In this workbook, we're going to start out by exploring what emotional eating is and its most common causes. We'll also explain how emotional eating is different (and similar) to an eating disorder, and why dieting doesn't address the problem at its root. When you're ready to tackle your emotional eating, the first steps are to learn how to acknowledge and accept your feelings, and identify your emotional eating triggers. We'll then get into the specific emotions that drive emotional eating habits: boredom, stress, anger, and depression. Throughout the chapters, you'll find lots of journaling ideas, exercises, and practices that help you deal with the feelings behind your eating habits.

To close out the book, you'll find tips on managing your emotional life and features of a healthy relationship with food. There's also an appendix with journal prompts and all the exercises listed for quicker reference.

You don't have to feel like food is your only comfort. Emotions can be addressed in much better ways and you can have a healthy, happy life where you enjoy food, but in its rightful place.

Chapter 1: What Is Emotional Eating?

As humans, we are emotional. Our decisions are often driven by emotions and that's not necessarily a bad thing. We also have emotional attachments to food. Fond memories of family and friends can be triggered by just a whiff of a fresh-baked cookie or a roasting turkey, while we're repelled by certain foods because of their association with an unpleasant memory. In that sense, all eating is emotional, but in this chapter, we're focused on how "emotional eating" can represent an unhealthy relationship to food.

Physical vs. emotional hunger

When we get hungry, we eat. That's not new information. However, when we eat in response to our emotions, there's something else going on that's not physical hunger. Food becomes a coping mechanism to deflect or soothe emotions we don't know how to handle. While physical hunger comes on naturally over time (or after exercise and the burning of calories), emotional hunger is swift. We encounter some kind of trigger and bam! We want food. When we eat, we feel better.

However, that comforting effect is always temporary and you're still left with all of the emotions that triggered the emotional eating. Usually, there are now more emotions piled on top, like guilt and shame. Physical hunger is satisfied after you've eaten, but emotional hunger doesn't go away and trying to soothe it with food can actually make it worse. Emotional eating is a vicious cycle.

The brain chemistry behind emotional eating

Struggling with emotional eating isn't simply an issue with will power. The brain is actually directly involved. When we eat, the brain is wired to "reward" us with feelings of contentment and happiness. This is so we will repeat this behavior and stay alive. However, there's a dark side to this natural process when it comes to emotions. When you eat in response to emotions, it triggers that reward system in the brain, so when we feel emotions again later, the brain tells us, "Food will help!"

The chemicals at play are serotonin and dopamine. When we get stressed, serotonin decreases, and we feel depressed and overwhelmed. Dopamine, another neurotransmitter, increases in response to food. While emotional eating isn't necessarily about what you're eating, more often than not emotional eaters are drawn to unhealthy foods high in sugar, salt, and fat. Why? "Junk" food has a powerful effect on the brain and the chemicals (like serotonin and dopamine) in charge of regulating your mood. Eating junk brews up feelings of happiness and contentment, so people usually seek out specifically-junky foods for comfort.

Symptoms of emotional eating

First off, everyone will respond to emotions with eating at some point. That in itself isn't a problem. However, if it becomes your go-to method for emotional management, it can become a problem. You develop an unhealthy relationship with food that's more consistent and persistent than just a weekly indulgence after a hard day. Here are some signs that you're an emotional eater:

You eat when you aren't hungry or when you're full

You reward yourself with food

You often eat until you're so full, it hurts

Food makes you feel safe

When food is around, you feel powerless to resist it

You eat to calm yourself down

You eat when you're sad

You eat when you're angry

The more stressed you are, the more you eat

What causes emotional eating?

Where does emotional eating come from? Everyone is different, so what triggers their root reasons and patterns of emotional eating can vary. These causes can include:

Boredom

Sometimes emotional eating can be triggered by a feeling as simple as sheer boredom. People frequently don't have the energy or motivation to do anything else, so they open up the fridge or pantry. It's a quick (though temporary) solution to boredom that can easily develop into a habit.

Stress

One of the most common reasons for emotional eating, stress can aggravate a powerful need to eat. When someone becomes stressed, adrenaline levels rise, and this actually dampens appetite. However, if the stress continues, the body starts making cortisol in high amounts. Cortisol triggers cravings and an increased appetite. When you eat in response, especially "junk" foods that give a burst of energy and happy feelings, you will feel less stressed. In that sense, emotional eating is technically working, but it can come with negative consequences if you're frequently stressed out and not able to manage it with other methods. People with anxiety disorders are often emotional eaters.

Anger

Emotional eating in response to anger may seem a little odd, but it's actually very common. Anger is often repressed because most people don't know how to deal with it in a healthy way, so food becomes the preferred way to soothe the confusion inside. Anger can also provoke a person into saying or doing something they regret, so they eat to numb the guilt and shame.

Sadness and depression

Nobody likes feeling sad. When someone has depression, sadness is a very familiar feeling. Unhealthy foods are often best at tricking the brain into happiness or at least a numbed state, so when those negative emotions appear again, a person will feel cravings. Even if someone doesn't have clinical depression, it's common to manage feelings of sadness with food.

Habits from childhood

Emotional eating frequently stems from childhood. Some people never had a healthy relationship with food and eating. Maybe their parents used the giving or deprivation of food as a reward or punishment, or in moments of pain and stress, they would seek out food. If these habits and worldviews aren't replaced by other methods of emotional management, emotional eating carries into adulthood.

Consequences of emotional eating

When emotional eating is persistent and consistent, there are a handful of potentially-harmful consequences, such as:

Nausea and digestive issues

When you eat when you don't need to, or eat even when you're full, your body suffers. Eating too much and/or eating foods that aren't good for you can lead to nausea, stomach aches, and other digestive problems.

Guilt and shame

Guilt and shame are very common for emotional eaters. They are often aware they have an unhealthy relationship to food, but feel powerless. Whenever they succumb to an emotional eating episode, their feelings of safety and comfort quickly dissolve, and they're left feeling guilty. This can lead to more emotional eating. This pattern leaves a person in a near-constant state of distress.

Long-term health problems

Because emotional eating tends to center on "junk" food, long-term health problems can arise. Eating too much salt, sugar, fat, and not getting enough nutrients from healthy foods can lead to heart problems, fatigue, diabetes, and more.

Poor body image

A common result of emotional eating is weight gain. This can have a negative effect on a person's body image. Looking in the mirror, going shopping for clothes, dating, and more can become challenging.

Low self-esteem

When you take into account the effects we've listed above, they all easily accumulate into low self-esteem. Low self-esteem can impact every area of your life from your relationships to your job to your hope for the future. Low self-esteem can kick off a torrent of negative emotions, driving emotional eating even more. People with chronic low self-esteem are also more vulnerable to mental health problems and addictions.

Eating disorders

Emotional eating can progress to an eating disorder. Emotional eaters sometimes go through cycles of binging and purging, which is a type of eating disorder. They might not purge, simply binge, which is known as Binge Eating disorder. Signs you might have this disorder include an inability to control how much you're eating, frequently eating even after you feel full, eating food very quickly, and feeling guilty and ashamed at the amount you're eating.

How emotional eating differs from eating disorders

Is emotional eating an eating disorder like anorexia or bulimia? Technically, no. Emotional eating can have an impact on your weight, health, and happiness, but it is generally not considered as serious as an eating disorder. Eating disorders usually have significantly more serious consequences both physically and mentally. That doesn't mean there isn't overlap. Emotional eaters are more vulnerable to eating disorders and emotions do play a big role in eating disorders.

Not sure if you're an emotional eater or dealing with a more serious eating disorder? According to Dr. Julie Friedman, director of the Binge Eating Treatment and Recovery Program, signs of disordered eating include persistently talking and thinking about food or eating; significant weight changes; an obsession with weight; and doing food-related behaviors in secret. Here are some more details on two specific types of eating disorders, so you can see if any of them describe you or anyone you know:

Anorexia nervosa

A potentially life-threatening disorder defined by avoiding food to the point of starvation. Symptoms include extreme weight loss, an intense fear of weight gain, body dysmorphia, and obsession with food and calories. Consequences of anorexia can include loss of mental capabilities, a higher risk for suicidal thoughts, depression, insomnia, irritability, and serious physical health problems.

Bulimia nervosa

A potentially life-threatening disorder defined by a cycle of binging and purging. Symptoms include frequently eating large amounts of food and then feeling panic about the amount; purging such as vomiting, using laxatives, and other meditations; excessive exercise; fasting; and body dysmorphia. Consequences include an increased risk for suicide, acid reflux, inflammation in the throat, dehydration, and heart failure.

Chapter 2: Why Dieting Doesn't Fix Emotional Eating

Many emotional eaters try dieting to deal with the consequences of their problem, but that only addresses the consequences of emotional eating and not the cause. Emotional eating is not something that most diets deal with. In this chapter, we're going to talk about diets, why they aren't necessarily a good idea for anyone, and why they are especially not a good way to manage emotional eating.

Why diets don't work

People go on diets for a variety of reasons, most often for weight loss, but studies consistently show dieting doesn't really work. Why? There are four main reasons:

Dieting makes overeating easy

When you restrict your diet, it simply makes food seem even more delicious and irresistible. The more restrictive the diet, the harder it becomes to avoid food and control yourself. In one study, 200 clinically-obese adults were randomly assigned one of two diets. One group had a low-carb diet with a 300-calorie breakfast. The other group ate a 600-calorie breakfast, which included a dessert. While in the first half of the study, both groups lost an average of 33 pounds, the group that got dessert kept losing weight in the next half. The first group actually regained a significant amount of weight. This suggests that restricting foods doesn't work in the long-term for weight loss. For someone with emotional eating, certain foods are especially tempting and restricting them will make them even more so.

Dieting can isolate you from others

When people diet, it can have a big effect on their social lives. Going out is a lot harder, so people often isolate themselves and become distant from their friends and family. While some social groups are willing to adjust, it's unlikely that will last a long time, because who wants to feel like they have to go on a diet with you? You don't want to feel like you're annoying your friends, either, so it becomes easier to just avoid those awkward situations altogether. For an emotional eater, this isolation can have devastating effects and drive their need for food even more.

Dieting triggers guilt

Loneliness is one possible emotional result of dieting, and so is guilt. Diets are built on doing things "the right way," and if you slip up, guilt will inevitably follow. The more restrictive the diet, the more guilt, because it's so easy to not follow every rule. Diets that use terminology like "clean eating" can also trigger powerful feelings of guilt and shame, because whenever you break a rule, you might feel like you're eating something "dirty." Guilt is a familiar emotion for people with emotional eating and most diets will just continue the pattern.

Dieting can be unhealthy

Many people, desperate for a change, will choose the most restrictive diet they can find. This is often because the diet claims fast results. However, restrictive diets are not only psychological tormenting, they can also lead to health problems. While there are diets that focus on whole, balanced eating, many of the most popular fad diets are restrictive and therefore risky. A restrictive diet cuts out an entire food group or multiple foods groups. The ketogenic diet is the most popular restrictive diet right now. The problem with cutting out so much food is that you risk micronutrient deficiency. Not getting the nutrients your body needs has consequences like fatigue, digestive issues, nausea, headaches, a weakened immune system, and more. This is bad news for anyone, emotional eaters or not.

What dieting misses

Most diets do not factor in emotions. When someone is an emotional eater, emotions are the things they need to focus on the most. Changing your diet doesn't actually change anything about your relationship to food, it simply swaps out one type of food for another. Even if you were to stick to a new diet's rules with a 100% success rate, the reasons behind your emotional eating remain. Eventually, they will catch up to you again, and you will most likely return to your old habits or just replace them with new ones.

Diets treat the symptoms, but not the cause. The only way to change your life, heal your relationship with food, and feel more in control is to dig into what's inside your mind and heart.

Note: While dieting won't solve your emotional eating, there is nothing inherently wrong with wanting to eat healthier while you figure out the deeper issues. Replacing your usual comfort food with healthier options does have lots of benefits, especially if you eat junk food frequently and are feeling the physical effects. By eating better, you will most likely have more energy to tackle your emotional eating.

Chapter 3: First Steps On Dealing With Emotional Eating

Deciding to tackle your emotional eating is a very brave decision. You are admitting to yourself that this is something you want to change, and you're committing to "getting into the weeds" with your feelings. In this chapter, we'll explore how to accept your feelings, identify what triggers your emotional eating habits, and prepare to shift your relationship with food. These steps are meant to ease you into a closer examination of your emotional eating, so you feel a bit more in control and aware of your body and mind.

Accepting your emotions

At the core of emotional eating, no matter what specific emotion triggers eating, is an inability to accept that emotion. Food becomes a way to distract and soothe, but it's a passive solution that doesn't actually acknowledge the emotion and respect it. When you commit to changing your ways, you need to commit to accepting your feelings. This is not an easy thing to do and it's something you will keep returning to. Everyone struggles with this, even if they aren't emotional eaters. It's a lifelong process, but it's worth it.

As an emotional eater, you eat your feelings rather than feel them. Emotions get pushed aside, buried, and hidden. There could be a variety of reasons why you do this. Maybe you were raised to believe that expressing emotions was a sign of weakness. Maybe you've had bad experiences in the past where showing your emotions resulted in dismissal or derision. Maybe you just don't know how to express your emotions in a way that doesn't make you feel terrible.

To stop your patterns of emotional eating, your emotions need to be accepted. There's no way around it. The first step is to get familiar with them and learn to recognize them. When you feel an urge to eat, decide to feel your emotions first. How do you do that? Here are some steps:

Stop, wait, and breathe

Emotional eating often consists of mindless eating where you eat without thinking about it. The first thing you need to do is just pause. This gives your mind and body a little time to sit in the emotion you're feeling. Rather than immediately distract from it or numb it with food, you make yourself feel something. Remember to breath. Really focus on breathing well - deeply and slowly. An urge to eat usually feels very urgent and deep breathing can help calm you down. We talk about breathing a lot in this book; it's an important piece of many of the exercises.

Ask yourself, "Am I hungry or thirsty?"

This first question is important, because not all eating is emotional, obviously. You do need to eat (and drink), so an urge to eat may actually be just your body telling you it's time. However, it often isn't because normal hunger pangs don't just hit you suddenly out of nowhere, so this question is meant to focus your attention on your physical body. If you don't feel physically hungry or thirsty, you know you're dealing with an emotion.

What am I feeling, overall?

Emotions can be tricky. You may not immediately be able to identify it, but right now, that's okay. You've acknowledged that you're feeling something and you know that you think food will help. To get a general idea of your overall state of emotion, keep waiting and breathing. Pay attention to what your physical body is feeling and any thoughts going through your mind. Are you nervous and jumpy? Or unmotivated and sluggish? When you take the time to pay attention to what the feeling behind the urge to eat, you will start to notice patterns and feel more in control. Those patterns are important for identifying your triggers.

Emotional eating triggers

What are triggers? These are the people, places, and things that bring on the emotions driving you to eat. Knowing what they are is very important to your journey. You may already have a pretty good idea of what triggers you, so take the time to get a journal and write them down. This is your "emotional eating diary," and it will be your best friend for the rest of the book. You can write down your favorite exercises, how you're feeling during this process, your hopes for the future, and more. Even if you don't think of yourself as a writer, do your best. This is only for your eyes. You aren't writing the next Pulitzer-winning novel. You don't even need to write in complete sentences. Decorate and doodle your journal however you like if that makes it more enjoyable, or keep it really minimalistic with just black pen or pencil. Some people like to just use a notes app on their phone. Whatever works for you.

Tracking your triggers

If you aren't sure what your triggers are, that's okay. Write down these questions in your journal:

Where am I right now and what's happening?

Why do I want this food?

If I eat this food, what will happen?

If I don't eat, what will happen?

If I did eat the food, how do I feel now?

Take your journal with you wherever you go. Whenever you experience an urge to eat, pause. Take a few deep breaths. Take out your journal and look at the questions you wrote down. Record your answers. When you've done this a few times, read over your responses and you will likely see patterns start to emerge. As an example, you might notice that an urge to eat arises when you first arrive at work. You are anxious about the day, and want to start it out on a happy note, so you eat. However, after eating, you always feel guilty and still anxious. Starting your work day is one of your triggers because it stresses you out. Other triggers might include:

Spending time with a certain person

Coming home after a long day at work

Going to a meeting

Talking to your mother on the phone

Being home alone in the evening

Having an argument with someone online

Looking at Instagram

You should also write down the emotions that accompany these triggers because those are what really cause your urges to eat.

Your life and the situations you encounter might change - you might get a new job you don't feel stressed about - but your emotions are always with you.

Anticipating your triggers

Identifying the situations/events helps you anticipate the emotions that will probably pop up, so you can feel better prepared to deal with them. In your journal at the beginning of the week (or the day, if you are a consistent journaler), write down the schedule you expect to have.

Think about what situations/events will most likely trigger your emotional eating. Be as specific as possible and also write down the emotions you think you might have. How will you respond instead of eating?

Changing your responses to triggers

As we continue through the book, there will be lots of exercises and practices you can do to replace emotional eating. As you read, write down the ones you want to try and plan on fitting them into your weekly or daily schedule.

How long until you see real change? Honestly, there's no one answer. It depends on a number of factors, like how frequent your emotional eating is, how many triggers you're dealing with, and how consistent you are with the exercises and working on your emotional awareness.

If we were to classify emotional eating and the exercises in this book as "habits," research says it takes more than 2 months to replace a habit with a new behavior, but that time frame can vary widely. For some people, it takes just over two weeks, while for others, it can take close to a year.

Next stop: learning to manage your emotions without food

Now that you know how to identify your emotions and triggers, it's time to really dig into what you can do about them. In the next chapters, we're getting into the most common emotions that trigger emotional eating, and exercises and practices that manage those emotions more effectively.

Chapter 4: Responding To Boredom

Oftentimes, emotional eating isn't driven by a big, scary emotion. You're just bored and you get into the habit of meandering over to the kitchen. It can happen so easily and so quickly, you eat without even thinking about if you're hungry or not. Boredom can also happen as a result of depression, which we'll talk about in more depth in another chapter. For now, boredom is a good emotion to launch into our exercises with because it doesn't require very much challenging introspection. What can you do if boredom is a big reason behind your emotional eating?

Ground yourself: are you physically hungry?

As always, the first thing you should do is ask yourself if you're physically hungry. A grounding exercise can help if you are frequently unsure of what your body feels. Grounding helps you bring you back to the present and out of your own head, which can trick you into believing you're hungry. Grounding is good for all emotional eating urges. Here are four exercises:

Reading backwards

If you have a book or magazine around, open it up a random place. Choose a paragraph and begin to read backwards. If there isn't a book or magazine around, but you have your phone, go to a website. Read a few paragraphs backwards. This forces you to really focus, and while you're reading, you aren't thinking about food. When you've finished reading, ask yourself if you're hungry again. Because your mind has been temporarily distracted, you're a bit more in touch with your physical feelings.

Water temperatures

When your mind keeps telling you "I need food," your body will begin to believe it. To flip the script, try an exercise that brings you more physical awareness. Running your hand under cold and then hot (not boiling) water can help. The temperature changes create a lot of physical sensations, distracting your mind.

Biting something sour

This jolting practice works if you have access to a lime, lemon, or another sour citrus fruit. Cut a slice and bite into it. You'll definitely feel back in your body with that sensation. After you've made a face and rinsed your mouth out with water, assess whether or not you're physically hungry or if you're feeling an emotion.

Drink a glass of water

Oftentimes when we think we're hungry, we're actually thirsty. When you feel an urge to eat, first drink a big glass of water. Pause and wait. What does your body feel now? Has the "hunger" been reduced at all or is it still singing in your head? Can you identify any emotions that might be driving your urge?

Occupy your mind with something else

Since boredom is one of the simpler emotions to deal with (on the surface, at least, chronic boredom is most likely a symptom of something else, like depression), managing it well isn't especially complicated The key is to actually commit to doing something besides eating once you know you're not truly hungry. Here are some ideas on what to do:

Write a list of 5 things

If you're bored and trying to resist an urge to eat, write a list of five things. What kinds of things? There are a lot of options:

Five things you can watch on TV

Five ways you can relax

Five people you can text or call

Five things you could read

Five games you could play

Now, choose one of those things to do. Keep your list. Hang it on the fridge, so when you find yourself standing in front of it, you have a list of other options to choose from.

Develop a hobby

If your life is not especially busy and you frequently find yourself bored, what are some specific things you can write on your lists? Starting a new hobby is a really great way to occupy your mind, so it doesn't automatically turn to food. When replacing emotional eating with a hobby, the hobby should be something you actually enjoy. If you're learning a brand-new skill or want to improve, check online for tutorials, guides, classes, and other resources that can help you stay on task and see progress.

Clean something

If you're bored at home, odds are there is some room that needs to be cleaned. When you feel tempted to raid the fridge, get into the cleaning supplies instead. Scrubbing the bathroom, picking up the bedroom, or vacuuming are all effective ways to occupy your mind and feel productive at the same time. Throw on a pair of headphones and listen to music or a podcast while you're at it for an additional mental distraction.

Is your "boredom" really just procrastination?

When a person is bored, it might be because they're putting off doing something else. To avoid doing that thing, they eat. If your boredom often springs from a lack of motivation, here are some ideas on what to do:

Consider why you're dragging your feet

There are often motivations beneath the surface when it comes to procrastination. It could be a fear of failure, a drive to be perfect, or low self-esteem. Maybe the task you're facing provokes stress, and you don't want to go down that road. Instead of eating, take a moment to access your emotions. Breathe deeply. Ask yourself questions like:

What am I afraid will happen if I do this task now?

Do I need this task to be done perfectly?

Do I feel like I am unable to do this task?

If so, why?

Sometimes, procrastination really does just boil down to, "Not feeling it." Maybe you're tired. If you decide your procrastination is not the result of some insecurities or fear, but just simply fatigue, commit to doing something (besides eating) that addresses that need directly, if you're able to. If you do need to motivate yourself and do the task now, read on.

Break the task into pieces

People who procrastinate are often overwhelmed by the tasks they have in front of them. It all seems like too much, so they put off starting it because they don't know when it will end. You can neutralize this problem by breaking every task into little pieces. This way, you begin chipping away at the task in very manageable chunks and before you know it, you've made a lot of progress.

As an example, you're at home and you have to start getting ready for houseguests that will be staying for a holiday weekend. Sit down with your journal and write down the different things you need to do, such as clean the spare room and bathroom, choose the meals, and plan some activities for everybody. Next, break down those things even further. Here's what the "cleaning the spare room and bathroom" task looks like broken down:

Clean spare room and bathroom

Vacuum floor

Wash sheets and pillowcases

Dust fan

Clean shower and toilet

Wash towels

Wipe down bathroom counter and mirror

By breaking down tasks into smaller pieces, you know exactly what needs to be done and you can quickly start crossing off items, which is motivating.

Go somewhere else for a little while

Sometimes all it takes is a change of scenery. If you're putting off a task and wandering around, thinking about eating, leave that environment and go somewhere else. This could be a quick trip, like going for a drive or a walk, and then returning to your task. If you can do your task somewhere else, consider doing that instead, so you are separated from the food that's enticing you.

Do something else for a little while

To stop procrastinating and get down to business, you need to get your engine running. Eating doesn't accomplish that, and usually comes with feelings of guilt and shame. If you're struggling with starting a task, just do something else for a little while that requires some effort. Read a book, do some stretching, clean something, or journal. Stop meandering around, because that aimless wandering is what will bring you back to food. By doing something, you wake up your brain and distract your mind from food so it can refocus.

Chapter 5: Dealing With Stress

Stress and anxiety are two of the most common triggers for emotional eating. Though they're often used interchangeably, there is a slight difference. Stress is something that everyone experiences at some points in their life and it can be triggered by change, difficult times at work, challenging relationships, and so on. Anxiety often refers to anxiety disorders, which are defined as more intense and persistent emotional responses to triggers. These triggers are often everyday situations. In this chapter, when we talk about "stress," we're also referring to anxiety because they can both trigger emotional eating.

What stress looks like

Everyone responds to their stress triggers a little differently. Symptoms are often both mental, emotional, and physical. They include:

Getting frustrated easily

Feeling down and discouraged

Experiencing low self-esteem

Not wanting to be around people

Feeling out of control

Feeling helpless

Feeling fatigued

Getting headaches

Getting digestive issues

Feeling sore and tense

Experiencing a rapid heartbeat

Experiencing low sexual desire

Not being able to sleep

Feeling shaky and nervous

Grinding your teeth

Always worrying

Forgetting things more frequently

Not being able to get organized

Not being able to focus or sit still

Relaxing exercises

If your emotional eating is triggered by stress, you are likely to feel a little better after indulging. However, that effect is temporary and you will probably feel bad about your decision. You want to replace your emotional eating with other calming rituals that don't come with negative side effects. Here are some ideas:

Deep breathing

When you feel an urge to eat in response to stress, engage in deep breathing. This is a very simple exercise that can be done just about anywhere. If you can, it helps to close your eyes so you are completely focused on your breath. Inhale deeply and slowly, pushing your stomach out, as if you were inflating a balloon. When it feels like you can't possibly hold more air in your lungs, slowly exhale, imagining you were deflating the balloon. While your mind will be tempted to wander back to food, keep returning your attention to your breathing. If you were experiencing symptoms like a fast heartbeat and shortness of breath, deep breathing should help. When you feel less stressed and more calm, the urge to eat should also be reduced.

Deep breathing is the most basic form of meditation, which has been shown to reduce stress. There are all kinds of meditation (most of these exercises are essentially different types) and the benefits become apparent quickly. According to one study, 10 minutes a day is all that's necessary to feel calmer throughout the rest of the day.

Object meditation

Speaking of meditation, there's another type that's good for beginners. It's a good choice if you aren't in a situation where you can close your eyes or if you need something else to focus on besides your breathing. Pick one thing in the room you're in and focus all your attention on it. You do still want to breathe slowly and deeply, so don't forget about that. Think about all the details on the object, like its color, shape, how the light and shadows fall on it, what it's texture might feel like, and so on. Do your best to ignore or even forget what the object is; pretend as if you've never seen anything like it before. When your mind starts to wander back to stress and food again, redirect your attention back to the object. Object meditation works as both a distracting and relaxing exercise.

Visualization

If deep breathing or staring at an object isn't up your alley, visualization is a good exercise. Instead of just breathing and focusing on that, you'll actually use your imagination to feel calm and peaceful. This exercise is easiest when you close your eyes, so if you're in public somewhere, find a place where you can be alone for a little while. Sit in a comfortable position and close your eyes. Picture a place or moment unrelated to food that makes you happy. Really think about what it feels like to be there. If it's outside, think about the temperature, if there's a breeze, and if the sun is out. What can you smell? What do you see? By taking yourself to a place where you feel happy and at rest, the anxiety symptoms are reduced and the need for food as comfort will dissipate. You're soothing an emotional need with your own imagination.

Progressive muscle relaxation

When you're experiencing stress, you might find yourself tense and jumpy. You believe that only food will help. Progressive muscle relaxation, also known as PMR, can be a good replacement. You can perform this exercise in full or in smaller increments, depending on where you are and how much stress you're dealing with. The full

PMR consists of tensing and relaxing all the muscle groups in your body, from your feet to your face. You tense each group for 4-10 seconds while holding your breath, and then when you're breathing out, you quickly relax the muscle group. Pause for 10-20 seconds between muscle groups.

There are sixteen muscle groups in total, so it may not be something you can do on a regular basis. In this case, take a moment to identify which muscle groups are most tense. Tense and relax just those groups and see how you feel.

Mindful eating

If your stress-triggered emotional eating is defined by frequent episodes of overeating, there's an exercise you can do to slow down and eat less. It's based on the idea of "mindfulness," which is just a term that means being present and in the moment. To eat mindfully, begin by first taking some deep breaths. After your first few bites, put down your utensils and chew slowly. Focus on what you're chewing - the flavors, the texture. Look at the food on your plate - the colors and shapes. When you've chewed your food thoroughly, have a few more bites. By making the effort to pause and focus, you're allowing your body to enjoy the food and it will be able to let you know when it's full. When you eat quickly and without thinking, lost in your emotions, you miss those signals.

Relaxing practices

We've talked about specific exercises that can help relieve stress, so now let's get into some other practices that can also help. These require less active steps or deep concentration, so they are a good choice if you're feeling tired and the idea of visualization or meditating doesn't appeal to you.

Reading

We talked about reading as a way to distract yourself, but it's also a good way to relax. Studies show that reading can be just as effective as taking a walk or listening to music when it comes to reducing symptoms of stress. When you're ready to relax, you don't need to worry about reading anything backwards. Pick something that's engaging and won't provoke more stress. As an example, it probably isn't a good idea to read a book about a chemical company poisoning a city. A relaxing book should ideally make you feel safe and happy.

Baths or showers

Warm water, especially in a bath where you're enveloped in it, is very soothing. Stress causes muscle contraction and heat loosens them. If your muscles are so tense that they're sore, hot water helps soothe that, too. Many cultures around the world have used baths as therapy for centuries, so there's clearly something to it. Studies also support baths as an effective method for stress relief. If you don't have a bath, a shower is a decent substitute. While you're in a bath or shower, breathe slowly and deeply. You are now basically meditating.

Aromatherapy and music

Smells and sounds are both very powerful when it comes to stress. The effects of aromatherapy and music have been studied for a while with evidence showing that they can reduce symptoms of stress and increase feelings of calmness. When you feel the urge to eat your emotions, light a scented candle or use a diffuser to fill the air with certain fragrances. Lavender, peppermint, and lemon are good choices, though any scent that makes you feel peaceful will work.

For music, choose something that makes you feel happy and relaxed. Certain genres are better than others; heavy metal doesn't fit the bill. Natural sounds like falling rain can also be very effective. Combine aromatherapy and music with a bath (maybe with a good book), and you have a fantastic recipe for relieving stress.

Chapter 6: Dealing With Anger

Anger is one of the most powerful and most misunderstood emotions we experience. Most people don't really know how to deal with anger in a healthy way. It's common to try and repress it, but it's also common to just unleash it without thinking. In this chapter, we're going to get into what anger is, its triggers and consequences, and how to deal with it in a way that doesn't involve emotional eating.

What is anger?

Anger is an emotion that can be triggered by a number of things such as feeling hurt or wronged. When things don't go the way we want or expected, anger can arise. Anger can be directed at specific people in response to something they've said or done, but it's also common for someone to just feel angry at everything. Feeling out of control or helpless is often at the root of anger. Most people think of anger as ranting and raving, but there are many symptoms, such as:

Feeling anxious and jumpy

Being quiet and withdrawn

Feeling depressed

Crying

Feeling guilty

Experiencing physical discomfort, like stomach cramps and headaches

Feeling dizzy

Feeling defensive

Anger shares a lot of symptoms with stress, especially when it isn't expressed. When it's expressed poorly, however, through hurtful arguments or even violence, there are other consequences, as well. Interestingly enough, women often have trouble identifying and expressing their anger, making anger a common - yet somewhat unacknowledged - trigger for emotional eating. This is no doubt because women are more socialized to hide and internalize this strong emotion, while men more often act out. However, many people of all genders can struggle with identifying and accepting their anger.

Understanding your anger

Like every emotion, anger wants to be understood. Anger is a sign from your mind that something needs to be addressed. While it's easy to just want to ignore it, bury it with food, or let it run free, anger needs to be analyzed and tracked for you to manage it well. You want to know the roots of your anger and its impact on your life. Bring out your journal and answer questions such as:

How was I feeling before I got angry?

What made me angry?

How angry did I feel on a scale of 1-10?

What was I thinking as I got angry?

What did I feel physically?

How did I react to that anger?

How did I feel about the reaction afterwards?

A few hours later, how did I feel?

Going through these questions in your journal can help you track triggers, responses, and impacts. You'll have a much firmer grasp on the things that make you angry and how your responses make you feel.

Exercises to help calm your anger

Anger can be an overwhelming emotion that's hard to control. It's like trying to get on a horse that is refusing to let you ride him. If you keep trying to deal with him (aka trying to deal with what's making you angry) without calming him down, you'll get bucked off. Discouraged, you then resort to feeding the horse/anger to soothe it, but it doesn't really help in the long-term. If your anger feels uncontrollable and unpredictable in this way, here are some exercises that can help you calm down a little first before figuring out how to respond to the emotion in a better way:

Come up with an acknowledge-and-accept mantra

To avoid eating your anger, you need to acknowledge and accept it. This doesn't mean you let it take control (we'll talk about healthy ways to express your anger in a little bit), but it does mean you acknowledge the emotion. This is an especially important exercise if you constantly deny that you're angry and try to stuff it down. That's what provokes a lot of emotional eating for people. Come up with a mantra that you recite back to yourself whenever you start getting upset about something. Here are some examples:

This (person/situation) has made me angry. I acknowledge that I am angry and I accept that this emotion is real and deserves my attention.

Anger, I acknowledge you, I accept you, and you will not make me do things I do not want to do.

I am feeling angry. I will treat myself with compassion, and I do not shame myself for feeling anger.

Anger, I recognize that you are here. I do not want to shame you, or deny you, but you do not own me. I will respond to you in a healthy way.

Write down your mantra in your journal seven times (this number traditionally represents completeness and wholeness) and commit it to memory. When you feel anger, write your mantra down again if you can, but if you don't have your journal with you or you're in the middle of something (like driving), recite it out loud or in your head. This process helps you feel more in control of the emotion and better prepared to deal with it in a healthy way.

Mantras may seem odd at first, but they've been around in some form or another for thousands of years. Studies show that this type of positive thinking has an effect on the mind and behavior, even if you don't fully believe it at the time. When you fill your mind with something positive, there isn't any more room for the negative.

Visualize a calming environment

We talked about visualization in the chapter on stress, but since symptoms of anger mimic symptoms of stress, it makes sense that this exercise would also work for anger. If you are struggling with controlling your anger and you feel like you're going to fall apart, visualizing yourself in a calm place can help. Go somewhere where you can be alone. Sit in a comfortable position and close your eyes. Try to breathe slowly and deeply. Imagine yourself in a place where you feel happy and calm. What do you see, smell, and hear? What are you feeling - the sun, a gust of wind, the texture of a warm blanket? Imagine as many details as you can, remembering to breathe.

Inevitably, your mind will try to wander back to what you're angry about, and that's okay. Be patient and keep returning to your happy place, imagining more details. The goal of this exercise isn't necessarily to get rid of your anger completely, it's just to calm yourself down enough so you can face the reason for your anger in a healthy way. If you find yourself ready to explode at somebody or ready to burst into tears in response to a situation, and all you want to do is eat, first find a quiet place and do some visualization. When you've calmed down a little, the urge to eat should be pacified. If you believe there's something else you need to do to address the reasons for your anger, you'll feel more ready after visualization, as well.

Write a Never-And-Always journal

When we're angry, we frequently think in absolutes like "never" and "always." This creates an extreme narrative in our minds that only revs up the anger, driving the urge to emotionally eat. Most of the time, that narrative doesn't really reflect reality. To deal with this false story and occupy your mind with something besides food, get out your journal. Write down what you're feeling, letting your anger direct your words. When you're done, take a look at what you've written and pick out all the extreme words you've used, like "never" and "always." Replace them with words like "sometimes." Read the entry again. Does your situation feel as overwhelming as it did before? Or do you feel a little calmer and less helpless? When you see the situation in a more realistic light, solutions can become clearer. The feeling of being out of control can lessen, along with the urge to eat.

Stop and listen

When you get worked up in an argument with somebody, it's easy to say things you immediately regret. To deal with the feelings of guilt and shame, you eat. However, if you could calm down while in the middle of a disagreement and prevent yourself from saying things you wish you hadn't, the urge to eat might not come up at all. The "stop and listen" exercise is very simple, though not necessarily easy depending on your personality. While arguing, keep telling yourself to stop talking and really listen to the other person. Focus on their words, body language, and other signs. Don't think about what you want to say next. Watch your breathing, as well, since anger will make you breathe shallowly and rapidly, accelerating your stress levels.

Sometimes it's clear that a conversation isn't going well even if you're doing your best to stop and listen. At this point, it's probably best to stop and walk away. Let the person know that you need some time to cool down before continuing. Do this when you notice your anger and stress levels are getting higher, and you know you'll want to eat in response.

Healthy ways to express anger

The exercises we just went over are meant to help you calm your anger, but oftentimes you do still need to express that emotion to manage it well. Many people see expressing anger as a bad thing, and they spend a lot of energy trying to numb that emotion, but expressing anger can be done in a healthy way. Here are some ideas:

Verbalize your anger to yourself

When you have a lot of angry thoughts racing through your head and you want to eat to quiet them down, it can help to just physically get them out of your body. You should be alone, so you can talk out loud to yourself without anyone hearing. Sit in a comfortable position. If you are mad at a specific person, imagine that person is sitting across from you. Let your anger out, telling the invisible person why you're upset and what you're feeling. If you frequently find yourself angry and you aren't quite sure why, verbalizing can really help you understand your emotions more. Sometimes, you might decide that you should actually talk to someone about your anger, so talking about it by yourself beforehand can help you figure out the best things to say.

Journal

Writing is another great way to express your anger safely. We talked about journaling already for the "never-and-always" exercise, but this time, you don't have to worry about that. Just let your anger out, spilling it on the page in all its raw, honest glory. However, it's important that you don't dwell on what you wrote. Reading the entry over and over again aggravate even more feelings of anger and stress, driving your need to eat. When you've written out your anger, consider ripping out the entry and throwing it away. Maybe burn it, if you want to be dramatic. This represents letting go after you've respected your emotions and let them be expressed.

Sing along with an emotional song

Music is one of the most powerful avenues for expressing emotion. When a song really hits you, it can feel like the singer or performer is speaking right to you and you don't feel alone. If you are at a loss about what to do with your anger and can't find your own words, find a song that fits your feelings and sing it out. If you're at home, taking a shower while you play music and sing can be very therapeutic. In the shower, most people feel safe enough to let their emotions out.

Move around

Anger can come with a jolt of adrenaline, raising your heart rate and making you feel antsy. Doing something physical and moving around can help address these feelings. Go for a fast walk or run around the block if you're able to. If you're not, find some pillows and go to a place where you can be alone. Punch the pillows, letting your anger flow out of your fists. Some people even scream into pillows to release the bottled-up angst tempting them to eat. These physical actions let you express your anger, but without hurting anyone else.

Say No to Food Addiction

As I've already said, when emotional eating gets out of hand, it can easily lead to food addiction. At this point you can't just help yourself. You look forward to your next "fix." Even when you are at work and it's not long after your lunch break, and you already had lunch fit for a Sumo wrestler, you start to get "the itch."

You may be wondering how possible it is to get "high" on food. Well, I already explained all that in the previous chapters. It's possible thanks to a hormone called dopamine, which gives you that rush when you eat. Ever moan or sigh when you eat something that tastes so good? That's that dopamine rush, coursing through you.

The Problem of Food Addiction

See it's not just about eating way too much at mealtimes. Food addiction involves eating more than you need, even when you're not hungry! This is where the problem lies. Say you've been able to identify you have a problem, and you've tried to quit. Then you fail. Don't beat up on yourself! The reason is you start to have withdrawal symptoms, since you're addicted. And since food is such a normal thing to have - unlike hard drugs - no one's going to try to stop you. Heck, you'll even find yourself justifying it. You've been good! You haven't eaten anything for like, three whole minutes! You've earned this pizza!

Food addiction arises when we eat for pleasure, rather than for sustenance. People who have that "sweet tooth" can relate a little too well to eating for pleasure. I'm one of said people. I will not deny it. It's just that I have over the years learned how to handle myself and my love for the sweet stuff.

When you reach for the sweets, you do so out of a craving for that rush of dopamine. You do it over and over and over, and not unlike with drug use, you start to need more sweets than in the beginning to feel the same high. Your body has come to expect it, and so you've simply got to deliver, or else it's going to throw a hissy fit by making you feel crappy.

So if you always end the day with a slice of chocolate cake, for instance, your body comes to expect that. It's become a habit. A routine. What happens when you don't give yourself that slice? Your body gets mad! But you don't even have to worry about that, because you've become so used to having a slice that you will find yourself unconsciously getting a slice even after committing to not doing that!

I have had people tell me sometimes, no other place will do except so-and-so store. They want their sweet treat from a particular place or store. All other chocolate cakes seem inferior, or just don't quite hit the spot right.

If you're this person, chances are you're addicted. When you decide to withdraw from the food, you get a reaction. Sometimes you get flu-like symptoms. There will be headaches, stomach upsets, and pure fatigue. Sometimes, you might not even realize that's what's going on. That's why a lot of people tend to feel like crap once they haven't had their morning shot of coffee. About 90 percent of Americans consume at least one cup of coffee a day, and 70 percent of these people can't start their day without one. A lot of people say they feel more alert and reinvigorated after a cup of Joe, and when they don't drink it the whole day seems to be difficult somehow. Many of them do not realize they are addicted!

Sometimes, you can get these withdrawal symptoms when you switch diets. Why is this key? You need to know so you don't quit when the symptoms come in.

Food Withdrawal

You see, it will take you about 2 weeks from when you start eating right to feel better. In the beginning of your new, improved, healthy way of eating, you'll feel like crap. You'll feel like you're currently unable to do it. And that's okay. Just wait it out. Trust the process. In a couple of weeks, you'll find yourself feeling better than you've felt in years. That's a guarantee. Reports show symptoms start to reduce after the first week, but you might feel very tired and drained for the first two weeks, or three if your addiction is that severe.

People do not understand the seriousness of food addiction because they can't seem to wrap their minds around how withdrawal from a simple thing like sugar should be associated with withdrawal from hard drugs like cocaine.

An addiction is an addiction. Your food addiction might not be as severe as withdrawing from drugs, but it is what it is. A positive change to your diet is very important regardless of the withdrawal symptoms you might have, because you will feel better for it.

It's NOT The Healthy Food Causing Your Symptoms!

A lot of people who have noticed they are having withdrawal symptoms think it is because of the foods or diets they are withdrawing from, when in reality it is the food changes to are making that cause the symptoms of withdrawal.

You can't just go from a mixed diet to an all-meat or all-greens plan; your body will show signs of confusion first, before you adapt.

Psychologists say experiments have shown food rich in carbs and processed sugar affect the brain the same way hard drugs like cocaine do, and so, suffering a modicum of withdrawal symptoms is perfectly normal.

This is the reason why people experience things like "sugar rush" because at that moment your brain lights up and your dopamine receptors go into overdrive, so you become alert and hyperactive. Doctors have found that sugar targets a person's basic pleasure and reward circuitry, this is what brings on the sugar rush, resulting in something akin to food addiction.

The amazing thing is symptoms of food withdrawal don't last long compared to withdrawal symptoms from hard drugs, which is a difficult and harrowing can even hasten the process of withdrawal by staying hydrated, eating olives and avocados process. You and drinking plant based milk like almond, soy, rice, etc.

There is still a lot of speculation on whether food addiction and withdrawal is "real," so, it would be wise not to take any drastic measures to deal with food addictions and emotional eating, because you might just be doing more harm than good. Here is a list of things expert dieticians and psychologists suggest when you feel you have a food addiction you are trying to withdraw from.

- Tread carefully

You need to be cautious and mindful of your withdrawal approach. If you rush headfirst into it, you might end up hurting yourself. It won't do for you to jump from one problem to another. It would be very unwise to cut off entire food groups at a go, especially macronutrients like carbohydrates, proteins, and fats. After all, the aim is having a balanced diet. Any slight mistake might plunge you head long into food imbalance. Results are better when withdrawal is done gradually, with a few indulgences here and there. Maybe a glass of wine on a special day, pizza with friends on a good weekend and so on.

- Seek help from a professional

Withdrawing from food addiction is not the same as withdrawing from alcohol or drug addiction, and does not even pose the same health risks. Still, it would be wise to seek professional help. It is important to talk to a dietitian or doctor about what you are planning to do so that you can share your concerns with them, and if they have any problems with your plan, they can put you through the proper way. They might recommend dietary supplements to make up for the reduced nutrients in your new course of action.

• Do not rush things

Some people expect a change in diet to make them feel better instantly. That is not usually the case. One has to first feel worse before getting better. It's the way of things. You know, "It's always darkest before the dawn." So instead of an abrupt cut, you could try steadily reducing the amount of calories you are trying to cut back on until you are left with very little or nothing.

A lot of people have noticed that after three weeks or more of steady withdrawal, they are almost unable to stomach the foods they used to abuse. Sugary confections taste even sweeter than they used to taste, while some foods can go as far as making you nauseated, especially really oily foods.

• Try a calculated approach

If you are withdrawing from sugary foods, you might have a really hard time of it. All your senses will willingly betray you. You feel like you smell chocolate everywhere. You could swear that book on your table looked like a piece of chocolate five minutes ago.

It's just a brown colored book!

It may seem like you are going crazy, but it won't last. You are just weaning yourself off of the sugar. If you know you will surely give in to temptation, then strategize, come up with different plans, and cross them out as you go until you find what works for you.

Planning ahead is very important. Clear your home and office of every tempting morsel of chocolate, make sure not to pass in front of the store where you usually buy your stash from. Include your friends and family in your strategy so they can help build your fortitude. It will be good for them too. If you find yourself in a place where everybody for some reason or the other is eating chocolate, run for your dear life!

Retreat! Retreat!

There is no shame in cowardice in this scenario. Be a healthy coward who has a low risk of having diabetes.

You could always find healthier food choices. I once suggested to a friend to cook something healthy and give it a chocolatey name. It might just work for you too. Why not try spinach sauce au chocolàt! Mind you, no real chocolates should be used. This is just a way of consoling yourself and getting your mind off things.

Coming up with a name could be very fun too!

Also try to surround yourself with people who are like minded or have the same plans that you do. It's a great way to make friends, and you all can find something to laugh about! Trust me, the whole experience can be very funny when you have people with a sense of humor to share it with.

Learn to Cook

It is important to learn how to cook. If you already do, good for you! if you don't, then invest in a recipe book. Because the reason a lot of withdrawals from food addiction don't work is that people that don't know how to cook, or are too lazy to cook, so they tend to fall back into take-out habits. And most of the choices they tend to make are usually unhealthy.

While withdrawing from food addiction, try to have fun creating healthier options for yourself. It makes the process a lot easier and takes your mind off of things, and before you know it, it's all over. Your food addiction a thing of the past.

Chapter 7: Dealing With Depression And Sadness

Depression and sadness are very common emotions, but many of us don't know how to deal with them. Everyone meets sadness at some point in their life, but depression is more persistent and serious. According to data from the World Health Organization in 2017, 300 million people around the world have depression. There's also seasonal depression, which affects around 5% of the American population, and postpartum depression, which 1 in 7 women experience. In this chapter, we're going to focus on depression and its symptoms as a cause for emotional eating because it is a more persistent problem than sadness. If you don't believe you have depression, but don't want to deal with normal sadness by eating, the exercises and practices will still apply.

What causes depression?

Anyone can suffer from depression, and no one is quite sure how it develops, but there are certain factors that make a person more vulnerable to depression, such as:

A past with physical, sexual, or emotional abuse

Conflicts with family and friends

Certain medications

Life events such as the death of a loved one

Life events that involve major change, even positive change

A family history of depression

Social isolation and challenges

Substance abuse

Other illnesses

Symptoms of depression

Depression looks like sadness in many ways, but there are some differences and the symptoms are more persistent. Interestingly enough, around 50% of people with depression also have anxiety, so those symptoms are often present as well. You might have depression if you notice signs such as:

Feeling sad during the day more often than not

Sleeping too much

Not sleeping enough

Feeling restless and irritable

Not being able to focus

Not having much energy or any energy at all

Not feeling motivated to do anything, even things you used to enjoy

Strong feelings of guilt

Low self-esteem

Numb or "blank" feelings

Not caring about anything

Engaging in (or thinking) about self-harm

Thinking about dying and death

Exercises to deal with immediate cravings

When you're feeling really down and craving comfort foods, there are other things you can do to address those emotions. These are meant for more immediate relief, so they work for both situational sadness and depression symptoms. In the next section, we'll talk about more long-term strategies for dealing with depression.

Watch (or listen to) something funny

Laughter can truly be the best medicine in many situations. If you are feeling sad and need soothing, put on a funny TV show or movie. For many people, watching something is still a passive activity and it won't help with their craving for food, so consider doing something else at the same time, like some light exercise, knitting, or coloring. If you listen to podcasts or audiobooks, choose a funny one and go for a walk. By focusing on something positive and entertaining, you distract from your cravings and bring some joy into your mind.

Listen to music

Speaking of listening to something, music can also be helpful in managing sadness and depression symptoms. It doesn't even have to be happy music. Evidence suggests that people with depression actually feel better after listening to sad music. This could be because hearing another person - the musician - express their own sad emotions makes the listener feel less alone. Music can also trigger tears, which release endorphins and oxytocin. Crying can be a very cleansing experience and many people feel better after a good cry.

Write a list of affirmations

When you're feeling sad or struggling through a depression episode, low self-esteem is very common. Your mind is full of disparaging, even cruel thoughts and feelings about yourself, and that drives your need for comfort food. When you're in a good mood, take the time to get out your journal and write a list of affirmations. This can be very simple one-sentence mantras or encouraging quotes you feel connected to it. Here are some examples:

I am worthy of love.

I deserve peace and stability.

In my imperfections, I am perfect.

Respect the process, healing is not a straight line.

I respect these feelings of sadness and grief, but they will not go on forever.

"In the middle of winter I at last realized that there was in me an invincible summer." - Albert Camus

"Just when the caterpillar thought her life was over, she became a butterfly." - Barbara Haines Howett

"There is hope, even when your brain tells you there isn't." - John Green

Affirmations may feel hollow and fake, especially during a time of sadness and depression, but studies show that dwelling on positivity actually affects the brain. Re-reading your affirmations, writing them out over and over again, and choosing not to wallow in your negative thoughts will have a positive impact on your life. They don't change your situation, but they can change your perspective.

Write a list of things you're grateful for

Studies show that gratitude can reduce symptoms of both depression and anxiety. Gratitude is a form of positivity, so it makes sense that spending time thinking about things you're thankful for can loosen the grip of negativity. When you're hit with depression-triggered cravings, take out your journal and write down what you're grateful for. They can be big or small things. If you don't have your journal with you, make your list in your head. Depending on the severity of your negative thoughts, this might be a challenging exercise, but really do your best. Keep adding to your list over time and re-read it when you're feeling down.

More long-term practices for managing depression-triggered eating

If you're dealing with more consistent, persistent depression and frequent emotional eating, there are more long-term practices you can integrate into your life. These should become habits and not just things you use to deal with cravings as they come up. The goal is to see real change on a deeper level.

Exercise

The motivation for exercise can be hard to find when you're depressed, but it's worth it. Studies show that consistent low-intensity exercise can improve your brain's ability to function. In people with depression, the hippocampus (the part that helps regulate mood) is actually smaller. When you exercise, you are helping that region's ability to grow nerve cells and relieve symptoms of depression. There are many other physical and mental benefits, as well. The best sort of exercise will be one that you enjoy, so if you hate running, don't try to run. Walking, using an elliptical or rebounder, swimming, yoga, Pilates, and more are all good options. Exercise can also help you manage your weight better, if weight gain from emotional eating has become a concern for you, and it can help distract you from cravings.

Build a social network

Depression makes a person feel like they are all alone and in our world today, detachment and isolation from others is on the rise, even as we become more "connected" thanks to technology. Everyone needs community and people they can rely on for emotional support. To help ease feelings of loneliness, make a commitment to strengthen and/or build a social network. Reach out to trusted friends and family and let them know what's going on. When you feel tempted to retreat into a cave and eat your feelings, text or call someone you know can help you feel better. If you don't have a lot of friendships or people you can depend on, start finding ways to connect with those around you. Volunteer somewhere or take a class in something that interests you. If going out a lot isn't an option for some reason, you can still build relationships online, though you should always exercise caution.

Go to the doctor

Depression can be very difficult to manage and sometimes you just don't have the motivation to do anything about it. You should strongly consider going to the doctor and talking about your options. Antidepressants will probably come up, and they are definitely something you should at least consider. Pills alone are not usually enough to treat depression and depression-triggered emotional eating, but they can provide enough support to help you deal with your situation better. In addition to talking to your doctor, it's a good idea to do some research on your own so you're fully aware of the side effects and if the antidepressant will be difficult to stop taking.

Go to therapy

This is probably the best long-term strategy you can take on when it comes to depression. Most experts will recommend therapy in addition to medication and it's common for people to choose therapy instead of pills. Therapy allows you to explore your depression on a deeper level with the guidance of a therapist. If you find yourself at a loss about what you're feeling and what to do - and worried that you're leaning on your friends and family too much - you probably should see a therapist. You'll be able to spill out all your feelings and receive advice from someone who's trained. Friends and family often don't know what to do and become overwhelmed. A good therapist will be understanding and non-judgmental.

Chapter 8: Tips On Managing Your Emotional Life

We've gone through specific emotions that drive emotional eating, but there are many other things you can do to manage your emotional life. No matter what triggers you, you can resist urges to eat your feelings and live a happier, healthier life. In this chapter, we'll go through some essential tips (some will be familiar already) and how they can improve your ability to handle your emotions.

Sleep better

Sleep is absolutely essential to good health. If you aren't getting enough sleep, anything else you do to try and manage your emotional eating won't be as effective. Not getting enough sleep comes with a host of other complications, as well, like a weaker immune system, a lack of focus and mental abilities, and a weaker heart. There are lots of things you can do to get better sleep and most of them are fairly simple. Here are some of the best ideas:

30 minutes before getting into bed, don't look at screens

Looking at screens (including your phone) stimulates your mind too much and can make it hard to relax and get to sleep. That's because the type of light emitted from screens actually disrupts the body's production of melatonin, a hormone that regulates your sleep/wake cycle. The body needs some time to "power down," and looking at screens prevents that from happening. At least 30 minutes before bedtime, stop looking at screens. If you want to do something before bed, read from a real book and not an e-reader.

Keep your room as dark as possible

Speaking of melatonin, the body produces it in darkness. The lack of light is a signal to your body that it's night - time to sleep - so it starts producing the hormone that helps you get to sleep. Keep your room as dark as possible to help facilitate this process. Move all electronics with their little lights into another room. If there's light streaming through your blinds, consider buying blackout curtains. You want it so dark, you can't see your hand in front of your face.

Use a sound machine or fan to help relax

Sound is a powerful thing, and if you have trouble relaxing at night because of stress or insomnia, sound can help. A fan is an easy way to get sound and a little cool air moving around the room.

There are also lots of sound machines that play tracks for falling rain, waves, and so on. Choose what works best for you.

Go to sleep (and wake up) on the same schedule every day

To build a consistent sleeping routine, you need to go to sleep and wake up at the same time each day. While many of us like to switch things up on the weekends - staying up late and sleeping in late - this disrupts the body's routine. In general, you want to make sure you're getting at least 8 hours of sleep a night. If you're sick, you'll need more. It's okay to break routine every once and a while for special occasions, but overall, you want a consistent sleep/wake schedule.

Eat well

It's no surprise that your eating habits matter when it comes to emotional eating and your overall health. What does eating well really mean, however? Here are two big things to remember:

Focus on balance, not restrictions

Diets don't work very well for emotional eaters. Restrictive diets don't work well for a lot of people. However, what you eat does matter, but instead of focusing on all the things you shouldn't eat, focus on balance. That means eating from a variety of food groups like vegetables, fruits, fats, proteins, and whole grains. You want to have the nutrition your body needs.

Eat mindfully

One of the best things you can do for your health is to eat mindfully. This means eating slowly and deliberately, focusing on the flavor and texture of a food. You are more likely to notice when you're full and not overeat. You are also more likely to really enjoy the experience.

Work out

Exercise does wonders for your mental and physical health. It can help address emotions that drive emotional eating like anxiety and depression, and help with weight management. Here are some ways to get into a regular exercise habit:

Do something you enjoy

The key to making exercise a habit is to do something you actually like. Don't try to keep up a workout just because it claims to be the most effective at burning fat or because you have friends who swear by it. If you don't actually like it, it's very likely you will just stop. Try out some different workouts until you find ones you enjoy, and keep those up.

Start small

If you don't work out much, trying to set a goal of an hour a day probably won't work too well. It's perfectly fine to start out small with just 10-15 minutes a few times a week and then build up from there. Everyone has a different schedule and aren't necessarily able to fit in hours of exercise a week, but that doesn't mean you shouldn't make a little exercise a priority.

Entertain yourself while you work out

A lot of people have trouble getting into an exercise routine simply because they get bored. If that describes you, make your exercise time more entertaining by listening to music, a podcast, or even watching TV. This gives your mind something to focus on.

Take time to just relax

Even if you don't have anxiety, it's very important to have times where you just relax and rest. When we're really busy, we don't get enough time to think about our emotional reactions to things and give our minds and bodies time to recharge. Here are some ways to do that:

Commit to a half hour of relaxing every day

Every day, no matter how busy you are, try to spend at least 30 minutes relaxing. It doesn't matter what time during the day you choose, but if you find yourself getting worked up or especially stressed, it's a good idea to take a break.

Meditate

Meditation is one of the best ways to reconnect with your mind and body. It's a very effective treatment for depression and anxiety, but it can help anyone feel more grounded. There's all kinds of meditation, so find the one that resonates the most.

Keep a list of ways to relax that don't involve food

Emotional eaters frequently relax with food in hand. To avoid returning to your old habits, write a list of ways to relax without food, such as baths, reading, drinking tea, and so on. Put it on your fridge so you see it all the time.

Connect with people

Community is essential to a person's wellbeing. It's very easy to get detached and disconnected, however, so make relationships a priority in your life. Here are three things to remember:

Be willing to be vulnerable

If you want fulfilling relationships, being vulnerable and open is important. It can be very challenging to put yourself out there, and depending on your history, you may have been burned before. Be willing to be vulnerable, but also be cautious. Don't open yourself to those you aren't sure are trustworthy. At the same time, though, don't hide behind walls.

End toxic relationships

If you have relationships in your life that bring pain instead of joy, end them. Signs of toxic relationships and friendships include jealousy, constant criticisms, unreliability, and unkindness. If you feel like you're doing all the work and becoming drained, it's another sign you should step back. Invest in relationships where there's mutual respect and positivity.

Go to a support group

Joining a support group is a great way to connect with others who understand what you're going through. There are all kinds of groups for depression, anxiety, and emotional eating through treatment centers and online.

Build your self-esteem

Most people struggle with their self-esteem, but if you're an emotional eater, odds are your self-esteem is pretty low.

Building it up is essential to living a happy life and having the confidence to manage your emotions in a healthy way. Here are ways to improve your self-esteem:

Go to therapy

For many people, their self-esteem is so low they can't improve it on their own. A therapist can provide much needed guidance and encouragement, even if you aren't diagnosed with any mental illnesses. If you really want to focus on your emotional eating, there are programs specifically designed to deal with the underlying issues. They are usually at least a few weeks.

Challenge your negative thoughts

When you have low self-esteem, negative thoughts frequently wash over you. Instead of just accepting them, challenge them. Push yourself to take a closer look at your thinking patterns. Imagine what you would say if a friend expressed those thoughts to you. You would probably try to say positive things to encourage them. Do that for yourself.

Be patient and compassionate

Building up low self-esteem can be a real challenge. For many people, they've never had good self-esteem. Be patient and compassionate with yourself. Accept that this is a process and it won't be linear. Sometimes, it may feel like you're going backwards, but that's okay. Don't berate yourself. Choose to be kind.

Have purpose in your life

The last tip for managing your emotional life is to have purpose. What are your dreams and goals? If you don't have any, it's easy to feel like you're just floating through life. Boredom, stress, sadness, and other negative emotions might be common. Here are some ways to get a stronger sense of purpose:

Do things that you love

There's a phrase that says you should do what you love. If you hate your job, think about leaving and finding something you're actually passionate about.

Spend some time exploring your options. If you are able to move on, that's great. However, for many people, that isn't possible. To make up for that, do things that you love in your spare time.

Think about your long-term goals

Do you have a 5-year plan? A 10-year plan? To get more purpose in your life, it's a good idea to think about the future. You'll have something specific to work towards and feel more in control of your life.

Plans can shift and circumstances change, but we can still dream and prepare.

Be generous and grateful

Volunteering your time and resources - and being grateful for what you have - are great ways to inject more meaning in your life.

These two things remind you of the bigger picture and help you connect more with the world. Your perspectives change and you'll realize how much of an impact you can make on the lives of others.

Dealing With Emotions

First and foremost, what are emotions?

Emotions are a state of the mind related to the nervous system. It is responsible for feelings of pleasure and displeasure, hurt or anger. Emotions are often mistaken for a person's mood, personality, temperament or disposition.

Emotions can be said to be the response or reaction to certain physical or psychological pressures that affect our behavior. They are a very complex concept. Studies show emotions affect a person's cognition. That is why it seems like people who are feeling some kind of strong emotion may not think properly at the time.

Identify Your Emotions

The first step in dealing with one's emotions is identification, figuring out what emotion you are feeling. Is it pain, anger, hurt or even happiness? Identifying what you are feeling is a very important step, because it's not so hard for you to deny your emotions, no matter how hard they stare you in the face. This is especially true if you're used to just shoving them aside, rather than processing them in a healthy way.

You could be seething with anger, but just choose to shove it aside, and claim you're fine. Or you could be sad, but you'd rather slap a happy face on, because it's more comfortable for you and everyone. What you're doing is wallowing in denial. When you can't express your emotions, guess what you do as an emotional eater? That's reach! Time to reach for the ol' bag o' chips again. Well, I'm writing this to help you beat that. Once you overcome that, you are ready to deal with your emotions!

It doesn't matter if you are feeling lonely, hurt, stressed, angry, or just plain anxious, it is very important for you to try to find some healthy ways of dealing with these painful emotions. A few emotions are a little less difficult to handle than others. When things start to get really bad, it sometimes feels hard to breathe or cope. Learning to cope with these feelings positively can help you live a healthy and happy life.

Let It Out!

Psychologists have found letting one's emotions out, physically, can go a long way to make that person feel better. If you have a lot of painful emotions bottled inside you, try to punch something - preferably something soft. No, not another human being.

Crying also helps. As does a long, loud scream. You could also jog or run. Or you could try doing what you enjoy, maybe singing, dancing, even playing a video game. Make a freestyle rap about whatever is bothering you. Write it out. Call up a friend and rant. Whatever you need. Just get it all out!

Once emotions are bottled in and suppressed, they become toxic. It is at times like this, when you're feeling emotionally low, that emotional eating is most likely to get the best of you. You know the drill. After you've eaten so much, so fast, you are then riddled by guilt or shame because of that short-lived sweet, sweet indulgence.

Finding A Solution

Once you have identified what you are feeling and have discovered what it means, then you can go ahead and find a solution. Take a moment to ask yourself if there is something you can do to solve the problem, Once your answer is affirmative, what do you do? Do it!

For example, if all your attempts at finding a job have proved fruitless, you could have your friends review and rewrite your resume. At that moment, if you feel there is absolutely nothing you can do, try finding out the best way to deal with that feeling of disappointment. Experts have suggested reading, swimming, writing, meditating, getting support from friends and family, exercising and seeking therapy.

Create Your Personal Emotional Toolkit

Consider these methods a toolkit. An emotional tool kit. You simply pick whatever tool it is you might need to deal with your emotions, and then make use of it. Whatever it is you need to use, it had better not be food, or that would completely defeat the purpose! Have you always wanted to learn a new language? Do that! Are you 35 and don't know how to ride a bike? Yay, something to do! Have you been meaning to write some naughty erotica? No time like the present!

Your toolkit could also be a literal toolkit. You should fill the bag with things like your diary, comics, magazines, your favorite music CDs, funny films, your favorite novels, inspirational books. NO COMFORT FOODS! NO foods, period.

Different Strokes, Different Folks

Different people have different strategies that work for them. It just depends on your kind of person, how you behave, how you interact with other people, and your ability to deal with your emotions. Your strategy might also vary from day to day! Today, you might want to hit a punching bag to deal with anger. Tomorrow, you might decide to meditate or go for a swim. The next, you might decide to listen to some amazing TED talks.

Mastery of Your Emotions

Emotions often feel overwhelming and intimidating, but taking control of them is usually the best way to deal with them. It may be difficult at first, but once you get the hang of it, it no longer seems so daunting.

Our emotions are like the powerhouse of our beings, as humans. Sometimes it's a good thing. Instead of us being as empty and automated like robots, our emotions push us and motivate us to be better than we are now. The issue is when we let ourselves become prisoners of these emotions. A lot of times, we let temporary emotions or feelings dictate or rule how we make decisions, even when it may lead to regrets in the future

Since most of what we feel and the emotions we go through happen almost instinctively, we have little or no control over how we feel at any given time.   But we can try to control how those feelings make us react, by taking the driver's seat on our thoughts.

To be able to interact well, and relate with people, we have to be able to know how people feel too. Because our emotions are the way we speak without actually speaking, without words. There are a lot of ways we can use to tell how other people are feeling, but usually by listening to what they say, and the way they act, most especially their body language.

Experts propose that a little over 80% of human interaction is non-verbal, which means it is usually by body language and facial expression. A lot of people don't like to talk about how they feel if the sense others are going to be affected by what they have to say. So their feelings tend to be more expressed in their body language.

The Limbic System

Emotions are unconscious acts managed by the limbic system of the brain. Scientists say this part of the human brain has evolved continuously from early on in human life, which makes it very primitive. This is why our emotional responses are always quite straightforward, but very strong and hard to control. This is because these responses are always controlled by our need to survive.

For a very long time, emotions have been strongly connected to experience and memory. If you have previously suffered a bad experience, your emotional reaction to the same or a similar experience is likely to be just as intense as when you first had the experience.

In that vein, the very first time you were hurt, or something bad (or good!) happened to you, you may have chosen to eat something, just because of how you felt. Now, your brain will have made the connection on your behalf. Anytime something similar to that event happens, you're inclined to do as you did back then. You're inclined to eat! See how this works?

Emotions and Values

Emotions also have a lot to do with a person's values. A person's emotional response can lead you to understand how they feel about something. The way a man might speak about a particular football team can make you understand what his take is on the team. You can even tell if a person likes another person by the way they speak about that person.

Our emotions are the megaphones of our hearts!

Trying to understand this association between our emotions and experience or memory and values gives us the key to controlling our emotional responses. Our emotional responses don't always have to do with whatever we might be going through presently, or what we are thinking about, but by observing your reactions, you may be able to put your emotions in check.

You have to take some time to observe your emotions, the accompanying reactions, and the triggers - be they your values, memories or experiences. Also put into consideration what experiences or values bring about positive emotions, and which ones bring negative ones.

Emotional Distraction Methods

There have been a lot of findings, writings, even suggestions on how to deal with ones emotions. There are a myriad of actions one can take that will be very helpful in dealing with one's emotions. A lot them are very common, but you have to try them to see if they work for you.

Distract yourself.Yes, it's really necessary. You really, really have to do this. If you are just recovering from a breakup, be proactive about making yourself feel better. Call up a friend and have them tell you all the reasons why you're such a catch! Get a great lineup of comedy shows and movies and prepare to laugh your butt off! Do it just because you deserve some joy in your life. Read a novel, something fascinating or intriguing, or go through a fashion magazine, see what is hot right now, and figure out how you can make it work for you! Learn a new skill from YouTube, or Udemy, or just do whatever will make you happy and keep you distracted! Before you even know it, time has gone by, you have started to feel better. That problem already feels inconsequential.

Exercise whenever you can.A lot of people have found they have been able to deal with anger or hurt by exercising, whether mildly or vigorously. Some have said they even go as far as imagining the face of the person who hurt or provoked them, while hitting a punching bag. It may seem a bit crude or violent but it helps! Exercise releases "feel good" chemicals in the brain such as dopamine, the dope chemical, which makes you feel better. Pretty dope, right? Being fit also makes look and feel healthier, which helps in dealing with one's emotions. It's either this or indulging in comfort foods. I am sure we now understand that emotional eating can be very bad!

Be thankful for the little things. Appreciate people when they do nice things for you, preferably in person, and try not to forget it. Be thankful for the clothes you have, the roof over your head, the fact that you're not starving. Be thankful for the weather, rain or shine. Be thankful for all sorts of things, and people!

Have fun!Having fun means doing things you enjoy. Do things that make you happy. Do things that are good for you and have no adverse effect on your health. Just have fun! The more you seek it out, the more it will seek you out!

Build relationships with others.Interacting with others stops you from always worrying about yourself. Open up to people, make friends, trust a little. Try to be grateful for the little moments of goodness and avoid unnecessary criticism others and yourself, no matter the situation. Always be mindful of your surroundings, and watch what you say to others. Don't you purposely hurt another person's feelings, because in the long run it may come back to bite you in the ass. Talk to someone. It feels good to talk to someone who listens. Spend time with people, doing things that make you both happy. You will be better off for it. You even feel happier because it will take your mind of some personal issues.

Don't give in to negative thinking. If you find you ever find yourself drowning in negative thoughts, then push yourself to overcome them, swim to the surface, get some much needed air and swim to shore. Never let yourself be pulled back in. Go for a walk outside. Inhale deeply and breathe in some fresh air, close your eyes and feel yourself breaking out from whatever negative contraction is around you. Take beautiful Mother Nature in. Notice the greens of the leaves, the chirping of the birds. Realize deeply and fully that you are not alone. It is very helpful in calming whatever raging emotions you might be feeling.

Psychologists have observed that a change of scenery goes a very long way in recovery. Go camping or hiking and clear your mind. Just have some fun! It's that simple! If you do not have the money to go hiking or camping or maybe go on a road trip, you could always go to places you know you will meet people you have never met before. You could go to the market, not necessarily to shop, but to be among new faces to distract yourself. You could go window shopping in the mall. Look for that beautiful shoe that you would love to get if you get enough money, then work out how to get the money to buy that beautiful shoe. It will give your mind something else to bother about.

Appreciate the good things in your life. Simply put, count your blessings! Yes, I've already talked about this, but it bears repeating! Someday soon, I will write a book about the sheer power of appreciation. It's amazing, and you will begin to see changes in your life once you learn to truly appreciate. Trust me on that.

If you can manage to balance your emotions, without hurting any other person's feelings in the process, then you have successfully learnt how to deal with your emotions.

Chapter 9: What Healthy Relationships With Food Look Like

In this last chapter, let's ask ourselves a question: what does a healthy relationship with food actually look like? You know that emotional eating reflects a disrupted relationship, so how do you know when you're seeing food through a healthy perspective? Let's go over the major signs that your relationship with food has been transformed.

You know the difference between physical and emotional hunger

This is one of the most significant signs you have a healthy relationship with food. People who can tell the difference between physical hunger and the need for nutrients versus an emotional urge to eat are able to deal with emotional eating. They can listen to their bodies, recognizing signs of physical hunger and thirst. They will know it's time to address that need with food or water. However, they can also recognize when their emotions are in the driver's seat, triggering a need for comfort. They won't be confused about they need food or something else.

You're able to exercise balance

People who have healthy relationships with food aren't obsessed with diets and restrictions. They are less likely to see food as "clean" or "dirty," but recognize the value in every kind of food. Instead of counting calories or giving food labels, they are able to exercise balance. Now, there are lots of people who have food restrictions based on health reasons, i.e. they're lactose intolerant. They can absolutely still have a healthy relationship with food. Food restrictions for the sake of control or weight loss, however, are not usually healthy or effective in the long-run. Multiple studies show that restricting food for non-medical reasons makes the food even harder to resist. You're more likely to binge on sweets when you're trying to avoid them completely. However, by using balance and including sweets in a diet full of nutritious foods like vegetables and whole grains, you will have a healthier relationship to food.

You're able to exercise moderation

Another key sign of a healthy relationship with food is moderation. This is similar to balance because it emphasizes stripping food of labels like "dirty" or "bad." Rather than trying not to eat any junk food at all, moderation allows you to eat everything you want, but in moderation. This also prevents eating too much or binging. Moderation is a sign that you're listening to your body and aware of what it feels like when it's satisfied.

You're flexible and forgiving

Everyone has some food rules and there's nothing inherently wrong with that. However, if the thought of breaking your rules (and actually breaking them) triggers a wave of guilt and shame, there's a problem. Your relationship with food and rigid rules are defining how you see yourself and your self-esteem. People who have a healthy relationship with food are flexible and forgiving with themselves. They're able to adapt to different situations such as holidays and social events, and give themselves a break. Even if it isn't a special occasion and they break a rule, they're able to move on. They don't struggle with a sense of failure or negative emotions like guilt afterwards, at least not for long.

You aren't ruled by the scale

It's very easy to get caught up in numbers on a scale. If you have a history with unhappiness about your weight, this has a big impact on your relationship with food. However, what the scale says doesn't have to mean that much in the long-run, in terms of your overall happiness and health. People with healthy relationships with food aren't obsessed with checking their weight.

Food makes you happy, but it isn't the only thing that makes you happy

It's impossible to not have some emotional attachments to food. It's part of what makes us human. Food should make us happy. However, we shouldn't depend on food for happiness and comfort. Food is just one thing in our lives that can bring us peace and joy, and in the long-term, it isn't the best source of happiness. When you acknowledge that there are other things that can help you manage your emotions and don't depend primarily on food, your relationship with food will improve significantly. Your brain will begin making other attachments, so when emotions come rushing in, food won't be the only thing you can think of.

Chapter 10: Which Food Does Our Body Need To Be Healthy

Eating a wide scope of sustenance that incorporate an assortment of supplements is the most straightforward approach to have a solid eating routine.

Here, you'll realize why your body needs every one of the accompanying supplements, and which nourishments you'll see them in:

• Proteins

• Carbohydrates

• Fats

• Vitamins and minerals

• Water

Proteins

Proteins give your body amino acids — the structure hinders that help your body's cells do the majority of their ordinary exercises. Proteins help your body fabricate new cells, fix old cells, make hormones and chemicals, and keep your insusceptible framework sound. On the off chance that you need more protein, your body takes more time to recuperate from disease and you're bound to become ill in any case.

During treatment for bosom malignant growth, a few people may require more protein than expected. Great wellsprings of protein are lean meat, fish, poultry, and low-fat dairy items, just as nuts, dried beans, peas, and lentils.

Carbohydrates

Carbohydrates give you fast vitality — they rapidly go into your blood as (glucose), which your body utilizes for fuel first, before transforming the remains into fat.

Natural products, vegetables, bread, pasta, grains, oat items, wafers, dried beans, peas, and lentils are for the most part great wellsprings of starches. A significant number of them are additionally great wellsprings of fiber, which your stomach related framework needs to remain sound.

Sugar (white and darker), nectar, and molasses are likewise starches. Be that as it may, these sorts of sugars are high in calories and don't offer some other advantages (like nutrients and minerals). Entire grains and foods grown from the ground are more beneficial wellsprings of starches than refined grains and sugars.

Fats

Fats give your body the unsaturated fats it needs to develop and to deliver new cells and hormones. Fat additionally encourages a few nutrients travel through your body. Vitamins A, D, E, and K are fat-solvent nutrients, which means they need some fat to be assimilated. They are likewise put away in the greasy tissues in your body and the liver. Fat additionally secures your organs against injury. Your body stores abundance calories as fat, which is set aside as hold vitality.

Fats give you more thought calories than sugars or proteins. As such, a teaspoon of fat will have a greater number of calories than a teaspoon of sugar or a teaspoon of protein.

There are three fundamental sorts of fats:

Immersed fats are found essentially in meat and entire milk items, or, at the end of the day, nourishments that originate from creatures. In any case, coconut oil and palm oil are immersed fats. Immersed fats are regularly strong at room temperature. Trans fats (additionally called trans-soaked fats or trans unsaturated fats) are framed when fluid vegetable oils experience a procedure called hydrogenation, in which hydrogen is added to make the oils progressively strong. Hydrogenated vegetable fats are utilized in sustenance handling since they give nourishments a more drawn out timeframe of realistic usability and an attractive taste, shape, and surface. Most of trans fat is found in shortening, stick (or hard) margarine, treats, saltines, nibble sustenance, broiled nourishments (counting fricasseed inexpensive food), doughnuts, baked goods, prepared products, and other handled sustenance made with or seared in part hydrogenated oils.

Monounsaturated and polyunsaturated fats are found essentially in plant nourishments, for example, vegetables, nuts, and grains, just as oils produced using these nuts and grains (canola, corn, soybean). Omega-3 and omega-6 unsaturated fats are polyunsaturated. Other than vegetables, nuts, and grains, omega-3 and omega-6 unsaturated fats are found in Coldwater fish, for example, fish, salmon, and mackerel. Mono and polyunsaturated fats may keep your triglyceride levels low. Triglycerides are a type of fat in your circulation system. Studies have connected high triglyceride levels to expanded danger of stroke and coronary illness.

Vitamins and minerals

Nutrients keep your bones solid, your vision clear and sharp, and your skin, nails, and hair sound and gleaming. Nutrients additionally help your body use vitality from the sustenance you eat.

Minerals are substance components that help control your body's procedures. Potassium, for instance, enables your nerves and muscles to work. Calcium enables your teeth and unresolved issues solid. Iron conveys oxygen to your cells.

On the off chance that you eat a decent diet with enough calories and protein, you're likely getting enough nutrients and minerals. In any case, in case you're accepting treatment for bosom malignant growth, this might be a test. Also, certain medicines may sap your body's provisions of certain nutrients or minerals.

It's likewise imperative to recall that there is a major contrast between getting your supplements through nourishment and taking enhancements (nutrients, minerals, and herbals/botanicals). Nutrients and minerals cooperate in your body in exceptionally complex ways, influencing each other's retention and handling and impacting how your body capacities. When you get your nutrients and minerals through eating sustenance, it is regularly simpler for your body to keep up an equalization of these supplements. When you take an enhancement, for example, a nutrient C or E tablet, you're getting an exceptionally focused portion that you would presumably never get from nourishment. While a few enhancements might be advantageous, others may diminish the adequacy of certain bosom malignancy medicines.

Water

Water is vital forever, which makes it essential for good wellbeing. Water makes up about half to 66% of your complete body weight. It manages your temperature, moves supplements through your body, and disposes of waste. Bosom malignancy treatment can once in a while cause looseness of the bowels or retching. Losing a ton of liquids in addition to the synthetic concoctions and minerals they contain can prompt drying out.

When all is said in done, it's a smart thought to drink 6 to 8 glasses of water multi day. On the off chance that you've lost liquids as a result of looseness of the bowels or retching, you have to supplant both the liquids and the fundamental fixings in them. Chicken or vegetable juices, tomato juice, organic product squeezes, and sports beverages, for example, Gatorade are instances of liquids that can enable you to supplant the nutrients and minerals your body has lost.

WAYS IN WHICH FOOD IMPROVES THE BODY

You have presumably heard consistently that you have to eat more products of the soil, more wholegrains and less prepared nourishment. Be that as it may, do you truly know why?

A ton of spotlight is put on the need to eat well so as to get thinner, and in light of current circumstances. In any case, there are numerous different advantages to eating healthy, other than weight reduction that you may not think a lot about. Nourishment contains supplements! These incorporate the major macronutrients protein, fat and starch (counting dietary fiber) and micronutrients, for example, nutrients and minerals. All macronutrients give vitality, estimated as kilojoules.

Let's step you through a portion of the fascinating reasons why it merits find out about nourishment!

1. Sustenance gives you vitality to traverse the day

Supplements called sugars are found in nourishments like wholegrain breads and oats, potato, rice and some dairy. Sugar is the fundamental fuel your body uses to keep the muscle and mind working. Starches are significant in such a case that you don't give your body fuel you come up short on vitality and after that can't do the majority of your preferred exercises in the day. This implies you would have no vitality to take a walk or run, do the shopping for food, cook suppers or take your children or pet to the recreation center. Fiber is an exceptionally mind-boggling type of sugar and it anticipates stoppage and diverticulitis and brings down your danger of gut disease.

2. Sustenance encourages us to fix muscle and construct DNA

Protein is another supplement that is significant for the body and it very well may be found in nourishments like meat and poultry, eggs, vegetables and nuts and seeds. Protein fabricates and fix muscles and body organs and tissues, similar to skin, hair and nails. Compounds that control the major metabolic procedures identified with processing, breathing and battling disease, are likewise produced using protein. Without protein, our bodies wouldn't almost certainly fix our muscles after exercise or assemble DNA which is our hereditary material we pass on to our kids and fixing it is a fundamental procedure for supporting life.

3. Sustenance can enable your body to protect itself and improve your wellbeing

Your body needs some put away fat so as to give protection and to ensure your crucial organs. Fat tissue is additionally a storage facility for fat dissolvable nutrients A, D, E and K. Fat contains unsaturated fats, some of which are fundamental. Unsaturated fats secure each body cell and help manage procedures like blood thickening and resistant capacity. Explicit unsaturated fats called mono-and polyunsaturated fats can bring down your hazard for coronary illness when they supplant immersed fats in your eating regimen. Monounsaturated fats can be found in sustenance like avocado, olive oil and almonds and polyunsaturated fats can be found in salmon, pecans and sunflower seeds. Expanding these sorts of fats and supplanting nourishments, for example, handled meats, including salami, cakes, take out and profoundly prepared sustenance can help improve your blood cholesterol levels by diminishing the LDL (awful) cholesterol) and expanding the HDL (great) cholesterol.

4. Sustenance can enable you to feel good, just as cause you to show up 'progressively alluring'

Nutrients and minerals are supplements required in modest quantities over a scope of metabolic procedures that work to keep the body solid, from breathing to deliver red platelets, to fixing itself, consuming vitality and battling contamination. At the point when these procedures function admirably, you feel better in yourself.

Nourishment, particularly brilliantly shaded foods grown from the ground, for example, carrots, broccoli and red capsicum, contain supplements called carotenoids. Research demonstrates that carotenoids can change the shade of your skin shading and give it a solid shine. Far better, is that exploration has demonstrated that expending the prescribed measures of brilliantly hued vegetables and natural product upgrades your skin shading to a point that others notice and think you look progressively appealing.

5. Food aids the brain.

There various supplements that might most likely improve mind work, which incorporates memory and consideration. Omega-3 unsaturated fats, found in pecans, canola and slick fish like salmon may help with saving or improving mind work. Late research is taking a look at whether curcumin, found in the curry flavor turmeric, and selenium, found in fish and nuts likewise help advance mind wellbeing.

NUTRIENT TYPES AND DIETARY INFORMATION

Nourishment is characterized as the admission of sustenance, considered in connection to the body's dietary needs. Great sustenance - a satisfactory, all around offset diet joined with normal physical action - is a foundation of good wellbeing. Poor sustenance can prompt decreased insusceptibility, expanded defenselessness to ailment, hindered physical and mental advancement, and diminished profitability. The eating routine of a life form is the thing that it eats, which is generally controlled by the accessibility, preparing and satisfactoriness of nourishments. A solid eating routine incorporates readiness of sustenance and capacity strategies that protect supplements from oxidation, warmth or draining, and that decrease danger of nourishment conceived sicknesses.

Eating a solid nutritious eating regimen has been appeared again and again to counteract an assortment of infections, including malignant growth. Great nourishment is fundamental to great wellbeing, ailment avoidance, and basic for solid development and improvement of youngsters and teenagers.

Supplement Classes

There are seven noteworthy classes of supplements: starches, fats, fiber, minerals, protein, nutrients, and water.

• Carbohydrates - our fundamental wellspring of vitality.

• Fats - one wellspring of vitality and significant in connection to fat dissolvable nutrients.

• Roughage (Fiber) - the stringy toxic part of our eating regimen basic to wellbeing of the stomach related framework.

• Minerals - those inorganic components happening in the body and which are basic to its ordinary capacities.

• Proteins - basic to development and fix of muscle and other body tissues.

• Vitamins - water and fat solvent nutrients assume significant jobs in numerous compound procedures in the body.

• Water - basic to typical body work - as a vehicle for conveying different supplements and in light of the fact that 60% of the human body is water.

These supplement classes can be ordered as either;

• Macronutrients (required in generally huge sums) - The large-scale supplements are starches, fats, fiber, proteins, and water.

• Micronutrients (required in littler amounts) - The small-scale supplements are minerals and nutrients.

The macronutrients (barring fiber and water) give vitality, which is estimated in Joules or kilo-calories (frequently just called Calories).

Sugars and proteins give 17 kJ (4 kcal) of vitality per gram, while fats give 37 kJ (9 kcal) per gram. Vitamins, minerals, fiber, and water don't give vitality, yet are important for different reasons.

The human body contains synthetic mixes, for example, water, sugars (sugar, starch, and fiber), amino acids (in proteins), unsaturated fats (in lipids), and nucleic acids (DNA and RNA). These mixes thusly comprise of components, for example, carbon, hydrogen, oxygen, nitrogen, phosphorus, calcium, iron, zinc, magnesium, manganese, etc. These substance mixes and components happen in different structures and mixes (for example hormones, nutrients, phospholipids, hydroxyapatite), both in the human body and in the plant and creature life forms that people eat.

Water is one of the most significant supplements in your eating routine. It takes out sustenance squander items in your body, manages body temperature during action, and helps digest nourishment.

Unsaturated fats

Most unsaturated fats are insignificant, which means the body can deliver them as required. Be that as it may, in people in any event two unsaturated fats are fundamental and must be incorporated into the eating regimen. A fitting parity of basic unsaturated fats, Omega-3 and omega-6 unsaturated fats, is significant for wellbeing. Both of these "omega" long-chain polyunsaturated unsaturated fats are substrates for a class of eicosanoids known as prostaglandins, which have jobs all through the human body.

Phytochemicals

A developing territory of intrigue is the impact upon human wellbeing of follow synthetic compounds, altogether called phytochemicals. These supplements are commonly found in consumable plants, particularly brilliant leafy foods, yet in addition different life forms including fish, green growth, and parasites.

The impacts of phytochemicals progressively endure thorough testing by conspicuous wellbeing associations. One of the chief classes of phytochemicals are polyphenol cancer prevention agents, synthetic substances which are known to give certain medical advantages to the cardiovascular framework and invulnerable framework. These synthetic compounds are known to down-manage the arrangement of responsive oxygen species, key synthetics in cardiovascular sickness.

Eat Nutritiously

Figuring out how to eat nutritiously isn't hard. The key is to:

- Drink heaps of water.

- Go simple on the salt, sugar, liquor, immersed fat and trans-fat.

- Eat an assortment of sustenance, including leafy foods, and entire grain items.

- Eat lean meats, poultry, fish, beans and low-fat dairy items.

HOW TO PLAN YOUR MEALS

It most likely doesn't astound you that in the present in a hurry, all day, every day world nibbling is a lifestyle. In the mid 1970's dinners made up 82% of grown-up calorie admission and tidbits contributed 18%. Quick forward to today, and dinners makes up 77% of calories while bites contribute 23%.1 An ongoing report demonstrated that solid, non-move working grown-ups eat a normal of 4.2 to 10.5 occasions per day.2 The main time <1% of the individuals overviewed don't eat is from 1am to 6am. Since the hours of day and night that we eat influence our body's circadian clock cadence, which manages all parts of digestion, dinner timing can have genuine ramifications for the advancement of cardiovascular sickness (CVD), type 2 diabetes, and obesity.1

The American Heart Association (AHA) as of late discharged a logical explanation that surveys the cardiometabolic wellbeing impacts of explicit eating designs: skipping breakfast, discontinuous fasting, number of days by day eating events, and timing of dinners and snacks.1 Here is the thing that they found:

BREAKFAST:

The AHA characterizes breakfast as the main feast of the day gobbled inside 2 hours of awakening, ordinarily somewhere close to 5am and 10am. Less grown-ups today have breakfast, which harmonizes with the expansion in obesity.1 Also, the Bogalusa Heart Study demonstrated that 74% of breakfast captains did not meet 66% of the Recommended Dietary Allowance for nutrients and minerals contrasted and 41% of the individuals who devoured breakfast.3 People who routinely skip breakfast are additionally bound to have higher glucose levels and expanded danger of creating type 2 diabetes, hypertension, and raised cholesterol levels. While there is a relationship between skipping breakfast and stoutness, having breakfast limitedly affects weight reduction, presumably in light of the fact that individuals today will in general eat various occasions for the duration of the day and the absolute every day calorie admission and sustenance decisions greater affect weight than breakfast alone.

TAKE AWAY IDEAS:

•   Fit a fair breakfast into your morning schedule with the goal that you expend a greater amount of the supplements fundamental to great wellbeing.

• For some, families, breakfast can be a fun time to eat together when nighttime's are occupied with after school exercises and different occasions

Have breakfast at work to save time at home

Pick a sound, adjusted supper for your regular drive: entire grain toast with nut spread and a bit of organic product is brisk, straightforward, heavenly and nutritious

Spare time by making breakfast the prior night:

• A smoothie with sans fat milk, plain Greek yogurt, or unflavored almond or soy milk; ½ cup new or solidified organic product, and 2 cups vegetables

• Appreciate medium-term cereal that you improve with natural product rather than sugar; include nuts or nut margarine for more protein

• Heat egg biscuits on your three-day weekend, solidify in individual segments, and rapidly warm on occupied work days

CHARACTERIZING LUNCH, DINNER AND SNACKS:

The AHA reasons that utilizing time of day to characterize lunch and supper isn't proper in light of the fact that there are such a large number of social differences.1 According to 2004 information from the Bureau of Labor Statistics, just about 15 million Americans work all day on night move, night move, turning shifts, or other boss organized sporadic timetables that effect feast timing.4 Is it 'lunch' on the off chance that somebody dozes during the day and eats their dinner at 12 PM? The AHA characterizes dinners as containing in any event 210 calories and any eating event with under 210 calories as a tidbit. Eating more dinners and less bites is related with more beneficial nourishment decisions that incorporate more organic product, vegetables, entire grains and lean protein sources.1

TAKE AWAY IDEAS:

Think 'smaller than expected dinner' rather than 'nibble' and you're bound to pick supplement thick sustenance, for example, natural product, vegetables, or entire grains rather than man made nourishments that are high in fat, sugar, salt and calories, for example, chips, vitality bars, treats and sweet.

• Rather than a vitality bar, pick a bit of natural product with nut margarine or 1 oz of nuts

• Rather than chips, pick plain popcorn, which is an entire grain

• Rather than treats, fulfill your sweet tooth with hand crafted trail blend that joins dried natural product (raisins, cranberries, apples, and so forth), nuts and seeds

• Plan dinners around vegetables, natural product, entire grains and wellsprings of protein regardless of what time of day you eat.

• Remaining sautéed food vegetables, dark colored rice and chicken or fish make a delightful dinner whenever

• Utilize your stewing pot to get ready suppers ahead of time that are prepared at whatever point you need a feast

DINNER FREQUENCY:

Is it better to eat three dinners for each day, or to eat a few little suppers and additionally snacks for the duration of the day? The AHA infers that there isn't sufficient proof to demonstrate that changing the occasions we eat significantly affects weight or CVD hazard factors, for example, circulatory strain, triglycerides, cholesterol, and glucose levels. The key isn't the occasions we eat, yet rather what we decide to eat.1 Consuming a by and large sound assortment of sustenance that incorporate natural products, vegetables, entire grains, and lean protein sources; and eating less prepared nourishments higher in sodium, fat and calories is an outstanding method to improve wellbeing, regardless of how often every day we eat.

TAKE AWAY IDEAS:

•   Focus on your body's craving signals for when to eat.

•   Abstain from eating since others are eating.

DINNER TIMING:

Eating late during the evening, characterized as inside 2 hours of hitting the sack, appears to expand CVD hazard. Individuals who work the 12 PM move and eat during times that a great many people are sleeping will in general have higher glucose, cholesterol and triglyceride levels. Interruption of circadian rhythms seems, by all accounts, to be at any rate halfway in charge of the expanded cardiovascular danger of eating late at night. The suggestion to eat like a ruler at breakfast, similar to a ruler at lunch, and like a poor person at supper may have logical legitimacy. A few investigations demonstrate that eating the biggest feast of the day later at night, rather than during the day, builds cardiometabolic hazard factors. Timing dinners and bites to fit inside 10-12 hours, for example, somewhere in the range of 6am and 6pm, may help advance weight reduction just as decline cardiovascular risk.1

TAKE AWAY IDEAS:

•	Quit eating after your night supper and rather remain caught up with doing fun exercises.

•	Rather than holding back on breakfast, make it the biggest feast of the day.

• Utilize a littler plate for your night dinner, and bundle the remains for a bigger lunch the next day.

CONCLUSION

The take home points summarized are:

• Plan suppers and snacks for explicit occasions for the duration of the day to oversee hunger.

• Farthest point dinners and snacks to a 10-12-hour time allotment during the day, abstaining from eating later at night. For instance, eat just somewhere in the range of 6am and 6pm, or somewhere in the range of 7am and 5pm.

• Pick dinners and bites that contain an assortment of supplement thick, sound nourishments as opposed to depending on bundled and handled nibble sustenance.

• Devour a bigger extent of calories prior in the day, making breakfast, lunch and daytime snacks higher in calories than supper and night snacks.

HOW TO LEARN FOOD EDUCATION

In the UK, there are countless people who need essential sustenance abilities and instruction. Individuals are uninformed of where their sustenance originates from and how it is created, what establishes a decent diet, and can't plan solid nourishment for themselves. For instance, a 2005 overview by the British Heart Foundation found that 37% of kids matured 8-14 did not realize that cheddar was produced using milk, and that 36% couldn't recognize the fundamental fixing in chips, with answers including oil, egg and apples.

Since cooking was removed the school educational program and moved toward becoming food innovation with the accentuation on planning nourishment pressing and sustenance preparing instead of preparing abilities and sustenance taking care of it isn't astounding numerous guardians get themselves unfit to cook. Jamie Oliver featured this issue in his Ministry of Food arrangement addition quote

There is a genuine peril that the present age of kids will grow up with no comprehension of where our nourishment originates from and without the aptitudes to pick and set up a sound eating routine.

A 1999 study by the NFU found that about portion of youngsters imagined that margarine originated from bovines, a third accepted that oranges developed in Britain and almost a quarter did not realize that the principle fixing in bread was flour. (Joanna Blythman (2006) Bad Food Britain. How a country demolished its hunger)

For what reason is this significant?

As a writing survey on educating of cooking aptitudes by Professor Martin Caraher from the Center for Food Policy at City University found that useful cooking abilities are crucial to guarantee comprehension of what establishes a sound life, and essential to guarantee that people can exercise authority over their eating regimen and nourishment consumption, regardless of whether by cooking and setting up their very own sustenance or by understanding the procedures that go into prepared arranged foods.

Prof. Caraher states that: Cooking aptitudes plan individuals to settle on decisions in a quick changing sustenance world. Without the abilities, decision and control are decreased and a reliance culture rises. Poor cooking aptitudes could be a boundary to enlarging sustenance decision in later life and therefore lessen the opportunity of eating steadily. In reality an examination from

Consumer Focus announced respondents on low salaries recognized the boundaries to a sound eating regimen as being too worn out to even think about cooking and not having the option to cook.

Caraher announced that various examinations have indicated expanded products of the soil utilization among kid and grown-up members in sustenance aptitudes clubs/classes. In spite of the fact that not many powerful examinations have been finished, nourishment abilities exercises do have a clear impact in improving the eating regimens of members.

Viable nourishment developing, through school nurseries or window boxes, fortifies educating about solid eating regimen, acquainting kids with new kinds of foods grown from the ground, and empowers open air movement and natural mindfulness. Jonathon Porritt, previous Chairman of the UK Sustainable Development Commission expresses that there is a real requirement for schools to react to ecological concerns, yet indicates creating nurseries and developing sustenance as one of the positive advances that can be taken by schools.

In 2005, a review by the British Heart Foundation found that 37% of youngsters matured 8-14 did not realize that cheddar was produced using milk, and that 36% couldn't distinguish the fundamental fixing in chips, with answers including oil, egg and apples. (Joanna Blythman (2006) Bad Food Britain. How a country demolished its craving)

What's the arrangement?

All schools should be built up their nourishment instruction. This will include all understudies having the chance to:

•   Participate in developing activities;

•   Visit nearby assignments/sustenance makers and homesteads;

•   Get the hang of cooking abilities;

•   Study nourishment and cultivating issues and think about worldwide points of view;

•   Partner with Personal and Social Health Education targets.

This will empower understudies to deliver solid dinners for themselves and families and thusly permit them genuine command over their weight control plans. In the long term it will likewise raise the sustenance IQ of the country.

A study by the British Potato Council found that 60% of younger students imagined that potatoes developed on trees. (Joanna Blythman (2006) Bad Food Britain. How a country destroyed its craving).

FUNDAMENTAL PRINCIPLES OF FOOD EDUCATION

Settling on the correct choices when you're going to make a feast is a significant part of your general wellbeing. We have gathered both the most sound and undesirable sustenance in unmistakably orchestrated records to make your life much simpler and better. Eating a plant-based, entire nourishment diet doesn't need to be confounded in the event that you need to simply adhere to the essentials.

Know that the sustenance to eat recorded underneath are a colossal determination of your various decisions – eat a decent assortment of what you like best and trial. There's no compelling reason to make luxurious dinners out of them, it's really a straightforward and local eating routine. How about we investigate!

FOODS TO EAT

Top off on solid staples first at whatever point you're eager

• Bananas, oranges, kiwi, apples, berries, figs, mangoes, pears, persimmons, papayas, peaches, lemons, fruits, melons, plums, apricots and so forth.

• Dried organic product like apricots, dates, apples, figs, raisins, cranberries, prunes, goji

• Fruit purée and other organic product purees

VEGETABLES

• Verdant green vegetables including kale, lettuce, collard greens, spinach

• Cruciferous vegetables, for example, cabbage, cauliflower, broccoli, Brussels grows

• Carrots, ringer peppers, leek, celery, eggplant, tomatoes, zucchini, fennel, asparagus, mushrooms, avocados

- Potatoes, sweet potatoes, yams, parsnips, beets, turnips

- Squashes like butternut, oak seed, pumpkin

Whole GRAINS

- Oats, grain, wheat, spelt, dark colored rice, white rice, rye, bulgur, quinoa, couscous, amaranth, corn, millet, buckwheat

- Items made of these entire grains like bread, sans oil saltines, tortilla, wraps, or pasta

VEGETABLES

- Lentils, peas, chickpeas, edamame

- Beans including kidney, mung, pinto, limes, soy and so forth.

FOODS TO ADD ON

Top your solid staples with these when you feel like it

FAT

• Nuts, for example, almonds, pecans, cashews, macadamia, hazelnut, walnuts, chestnuts, pine, coconut and so on.

• Seeds like flax, sunflower, sesame, chia and so on.

• Tahini, nut spread like almond margarine, cashew spread and so forth.

PROTEIN

• Plant-based milk produced using soy, rice, almonds, hazelnut, hemp

• Kefir, yogurt or cream made of the fixings above

• Tofu plain, smoked, or spiced however no phony meats, frankfurters or tofurky

CARBS

• Refined flour items like pasta, bread, soba rice noodles

• Cornflakes, sans sugar cold oat,

- Refined flours (rice, rye, wheat, oat, corn, buckwheat, grain)

Sauces and SPICES

- Common sugars, for example, date syrup or molasses, unadulterated sweetener, oak seed/maple syrup, date glue, stevia leaves, agave nectar

- Soy sauce, balsamic vinegar, apple juice vinegar, miso, hot sauce, ocean salt, vegetable stock, ketchup, sriracha, curry glue, tomato glue, dietary yeast

- Flavors like garlic, onion, new herbs (basil, parsley, rosemary, oregano, mint and so on), scallions, bean stew, cardamom, curry, ginger, mustard, pepper, cinnamon, coriander, vanilla, garam masala, nutmeg, turmeric and so on.

FOODS TO AVOID

Make sure to avoid these fixings when conceivable

- Every single ANIMAL Product

- Any sort of meat like hamburger, pork, poultry, turkey, sheep, game meat and so on.

- Fish, shellfish, eggs, and nourishment made with any of these like mayonnaise

•   Dairy milk and all nourishment made with them

•   Cheddar, cream cheddar, curds, sharp cream, yogurt, frozen yogurt, margarine

ALL OILS

•   Margarine and vegetable oils, for example, olive oil, coconut oil, sunflower oil, and fish oil and so on.

•   Items containing oils like spreads, treats, prepared merchandise, sauces and so on.

Profoundly PROCESSED FOODS

•   High fructose corn syrup, white sugar, nectar and nourishments made with them

•   Sugary grains, chocolate bars, pop, counterfeit sugars, doughnuts

HYDRATION

•   Drinking enough water ought to be guaranteed, regardless of what diet somebody eats. Contingent upon the temperature and how much action you're getting, attempt to drink in any event 1.5 – 2 liters of water multi day. Other potential drinks which you can add to your water are tea, espresso (on the off chance that you don't feel any reactions), and organic product or vegetable juices (natively constructed is ideal).

•	Pay special mind to great quality and don't get concentrates or anything with included sugar! Additionally, don't load up your tea or espresso with cream and sugar, choose some stevia with soy milk rather or drink it plain. Another thought is to make some organic product mixed water by putting a few cuts of citrus natural product or berries alongside new herbs like mint into a jug of water and after that drink it. Liquor won't help you also, so avoid it however much as could be expected.

GENERAL FOOD GUIDELINES

•	Consider foods 'high' or 'low' supplement thick and make progress toward most extreme sustenance

•	Eat the same number of entire sustenance as you need, include some insignificantly handled nourishments in to a great extent

- Tune in to your appetite and never starve yourself – eat until you're fulfilled however not stuffed

- Try not to disregard hydration, drink fundamentally unadulterated water just as natural product/vegetable juice when you feel like it (around 2-3 liters per day)

- Try not to fear carbs or entire fats, there is no compelling reason to tally macronutrients when eating an entire sustenance, plant-based eating regimen

- For whatever length of time that you meet your caloric needs, you can't get protein insufficient even on simply plant sustenance

- Both crude and cooked sustenance have various advantages so don't hesitate to devour them in the proportion that suits you best

- Attempt to get ready as much sustenance as you can at home and utilize without a doubt, almost no salt or sugar. Skirt the oil.

- Try not to get excessively extraordinary and attempt to be extremely 'unadulterated' by eating just green verdant vegetables, since it's unsustainable and uneven.

WHAT THE GUIDELINES ARE BASED ON CLEAN - Wash Hands Often

Combined with the significance of hand-washing, the Dietary Guidelines reminds customers to altogether wash all kitchen surfaces, including machines, reusable basic food item packs, and all produce (regardless of whether you intend to strip and cut before eating). For instance, the internal parts of microwaves frequently become dirtied with nourishment, enabling microscopic organisms to develop. By washing both within and outside, including handles and catches, food contamination might be averted.

• Legitimate hand-washing may take out a huge level of food contamination cases and fundamentally decrease the spread of the basic cold and influenza.

• Wash hands previously, during and after feast arrangement, subsequent to utilizing the washroom, in the wake of changing diapers and in the wake of dealing with pets and pet waste.

• Wash turns in warm, sudsy water for in any event 20 seconds.

• Remember to keep surfaces clean, including racks, ledges, tables, fridges and coolers.

Isolated - Keep Ready-to-Eat Foods Separate from Raw Meat Poultry, Seafood and Eggs

At the point when juices from crude meats or germs from unclean items unintentionally contact cooked or prepared to-eat sustenance, for example, products of the soil, cross-sullying happens.

• Anticipate cross-pollution by keeping crude meat, poultry, fish and eggs separate from prepared to-eat sustenance.

• Utilize two cuttings sheets: one carefully for crude meat, poultry and fish; the other for prepared to-eat nourishments including breads and vegetables.

• Wash cutting sheets completely in hot sudsy water after each utilization or spot in dishwasher. Utilize a sanitizer arrangement (one tablespoon fade in one-quart water) or other sterilizing arrangement and wash with clean water.

• Dispose of old cutting sheets that have splits, cleft and unnecessary blade scars.

CHILL - Refrigerate Promptly to 40 Degrees Fahrenheit or Below

• Refrigerate foods immediately and at a legitimate temperature to slow the development of microorganisms and anticipate food contamination.

• Ensure your fridge is set underneath 40°F and cooler is at or beneath 0°F.

• Keep a fridge thermometer in your icebox and check it normally.

• Refrigerate transient nourishment when you return home from the store.

• Refrigerate every extra nourishment from a feast inside two hours. Whenever outside and the temperature is 90°F or hotter, that time is diminished to 60 minutes.

• Store nourishments in little, shallow holders (two inches down or less).

• Use or dispose of opened bundles of lunch get-together meats or spreads inside three to five days. Devour by the "utilization by" date on the bundle.

• Defrost nourishment in the fridge, under virus running water, or in the microwave directly before cooking.

• Marinate sustenance in the fridge, not on the counter.

COOK - Cook to Proper Temperatures

• Fish, fish, meat, poultry and egg dishes ought to be cooked to the prescribed safe least inside temperature to decimate any conceivably hurtful microbes.

• Continuously utilize a sustenance thermometer to check the doneness of meat, poultry, fish and dishes containing eggs.

• Warm scraps to at any rate 165°F. More established grown-ups ought to warm all store style meats.

• Heat up a meat marinade for a few minutes in the event that you plan to re-use it.

Utilize the accompanying brisk interior temperature manage:

• Meat, veal, sheep 145°F (with 3 minutes of rest time)

- Pork 160°F

- Poultry 165°F

- Ground meat, veal, sheep 160°F

- Ground poultry 165°F

- Finfish 145°F or until tissue is obscure and pieces with a fork

- Shellfish cook until tissue is obscure all through

- Eggs yolk and white are firm, not runny

- Meals, egg dishes 165°F

- Remains 165°F; bubble fluids (soup, sauce)

DIALECTIC BEHAVIOUR THERAPY

Dialectic Behavior Therapy (DBT) is a kind of subjective social treatment. Its fundamental objectives are to show individuals how to live at the time, adapt soundly to pressure, manage feelings, and improve associations with others.

USE OF DBT

It was initially expected for individuals with marginal character issue however has since been adjusted for different conditions where the patient displays reckless conduct, for example, dietary issues and substance misuse. It is additionally here and there used to treat post-horrendous pressure issue.

HISTORY

DBT was created in the late 1980s by Dr. Marsha Linehan and associates when they found that intellectual conduct treatment alone did not function just as expected in patients with marginal character issue. Dr. Linehan and her group included strategies and built up a treatment which would meet the interesting needs of these patients.

DBT is gotten from a philosophical procedure called rationalizations. Arguments depends on the idea that everything is made out of contrary energies and that change happens when one restricting power is more grounded than the other, or in progressively scholastic terms—postulation, direct opposite, and blend.

All the more explicitly, rationalizations makes three essential suppositions:

- Everything is interconnected.

- Change is consistent and inescapable.

- Contrary energies can be coordinated to frame a closer estimate of reality.

Along these lines in DBT, the patient and specialist are attempting to determine the appearing inconsistency between self-acknowledgment and change so as to realize positive changes in the patient.

Another strategy offered by Linehan and her partners was approval. Linehan and her group found that with approval, alongside the push for change, patients were bound to collaborate and less inclined to endure trouble at change. The specialist approves that the individual's activities "bode well" inside the setting of his own encounters without fundamentally concurring that they are the best way to deal with taking care of the issue.

DBT as a Type of Cognitive Behavioral Therapy

DBT has now developed into a standard kind of subjective conduct treatment. At the point when an individual is experiencing DBT, they can hope to take part in three helpful settings:

A study hall where an individual is shown social abilities by doing schoolwork assignments and pretending better approaches for cooperating with individuals

Singular treatment with a prepared proficient where those scholarly conduct aptitudes are adjusted to an individual's close to home life challenges

Telephone training in which an individual can call their specialist to get direction on adapting to a troublesome right now circumstance

In DBT, singular specialists likewise meet with a discussion group to enable them to remain inspired in treating their patients and help them explore troublesome and complex issues.

Four Modules

Individuals experiencing DBT are encouraged how to viably change their conduct utilizing four fundamental methodologies:

- Care—concentrating on the present ("living at the time").

- Trouble Tolerance—figuring out how to acknowledge oneself and the present circumstance. All the more explicitly, individuals figure out how to endure or endure emergencies utilizing these four systems: diversion, self-relieving, improving the development, and considering upsides and downsides.

- Relational Effectiveness—how to be confident in a relationship (for instance, communicating needs and saying "no") yet at the same time keeping that relationship positive and solid.

- Feeling Regulation—perceiving and adapting to negative feelings (for instance, outrage) and decreasing one's passionate weakness by expanding positive emotional encounters.

Chapter 11: Don't Make The Same Mistake

COMMON MISCONCEPTIONS ABOUT EATING DISORDERS

While the greater part of us consider self-perception as an odd, ungainly subject, it is an issue that should be discussed. Nearly everybody needs to change parts of their physical appearance, yet for certain individuals, these wants can transform into a constant fixation on eating, weight reduction and exercise. The three primary dietary problems are Anorexia Nervosa (portrayed by definitely limiting caloric admission), Bulimia Nervosa (described by expending a lot of nourishments, at that point cleansing them by retching or through exercise), and Binge Eating Disorder, which resembles bulimia, without the cleansing.

While individuals may kid about expending extraordinary measures of nourishments on the double or attempting to be "ano," dietary issues are intense, and regularly excessively misjudged. To support your comprehension of dietary problems we have recorded 10 legends exposed that may change what you think.

Legend #1: People with dietary issues are vain

This is false. Usually, individuals who create dietary issues simply need to attempt another eating regimen to improve themselves and for a chosen few, this tragically can transform into wild maladies. This does not mean individuals with dietary issues are fixated on themselves or vain in any sense. Likewise, wretchedness, tension and temperament issue are amazingly basic for those with dietary issues, and more often than not they come to fruition as an approach to control different issues.

Fantasy #2: People have dietary issues. They simply need to wake up

Much the same as you wouldn't blame somebody for having asthma or malignancy, you shouldn't censure somebody for building up a dietary issue. Studies have shown that hereditary qualities represent up to 80% of the hazard for creating dietary problems.

Dietary issues are not kidding diseases with mental and physical results that regularly include a lot of affliction. Somebody can settle on the decision to seek after recuperation, yet the demonstration of recuperation itself is a ton of diligent work and includes more than essentially choosing to not follow up on side effects. As a rule, the dietary problem has turned into an individual's essential method for adapting to extraordinary feelings and troublesome life occasions. So as to recuperate from the dietary issue, an individual needs proper treatment and backing with respect to medicinal observing, wholesome recovery just as learning and rehearsing more beneficial approaches to oversee pressure.

Legend #3: People with anorexia should "simply eat" as of now

It might be difficult to understand how somebody could leave behind a plate of warm treats; however, anorexia actually changes the mind, making eating an alarming thing, and even blunts the taste buds. Sustenance is never again a wellspring of delight.

Fantasy #4: Eating issue aren't not kidding. They're only a stage

Anorexia is the #1 mental executioner, asserting a bigger number of unfortunate casualties than wretchedness and suicide. Anorexia and bulimia can for all time harm bones, regenerative wellbeing and every single significant organ including the heart and cerebrum.

Fantasy #5: Only young ladies can get dietary issues

False! In spite of the fact that they are most regular among school females, people everything being equal and ethnicities experience the ill effects of dietary problems and self-perception issues.

At any rate 1 out of each 10 individuals with a dietary problem is male. Truth be told, inside certain indicative classes like Binge Eating Disorder, men speak to the same number of as 40% of those influenced. In an as of late discharged report from the American Academy of Pediatrics, young men and men were referred to as one of the gatherings seeing the quickest ascent in dietary issues in the course of recent years alongside 8-multi year old and ethnic minorities. It's similarly imperative to screen for dietary problems among females and guys.

Legend #6: People who are anorexic never eat

Individuals with anorexia do eat. Nonetheless, they radically limit the measure of calories they can devour and regularly exercise like there's no tomorrow. What's most telling is the sentiments of nervousness and dread identified with controlling sustenance admission.

Fantasy #7: Binge Eating Disorder is certifiably not a genuine article

Everybody indulges. In any case, a few people feel like they can't control themselves and will stuff heaps of sustenance into their bodies in short measures of time and feel unfit to stop, regardless of whether they're full. This is a genuine issue and shouldn't be overlooked.

Fantasy #8: My companion is fixated on sustenance

It is extremely unlikely she can have a dietary issue.

In reality, a warning for a dietary problem is an abrupt, extraordinary fixation on sustenance, gathering plans and watching nourishment TV. The less nourishment they eat, the more they need to think about it.

Fantasy #9: I know somebody with extremely strange, over the top dietary patterns, yet they're not very thin, so they should be fine.

False once more! Regardless of whether somebody isn't perilously underweight, they may even now have an ailment that requirements treatment. What's more, since bulimics don't cleanse the vast majority of the calories they devour, they are regularly of ordinary weight or may even increase a few.

Fantasy #10: Eating issue are cumbersome to discuss so it's fine to disregard them

While its actual dietary problems are a tricky subject to examine, on the off chance that you or somebody you know has signs or manifestations of scattered eating conduct, shouting out is the initial move towards getting more joyful and more advantageous.

LEARN HEALTHY MEAL PREPARATION

Arranging an everyday menu isn't troublesome as long as every supper and tidbit have some protein, fiber, complex sugars and a tad of fat. This is what you have to think about every dinner.

• Having breakfast will enable you to begin your day with a lot of vitality. Try not to destroy your morning meal with high-fat and unhealthy sustenance. Pick some protein and fiber for your morning meal, and it's a decent time to eat some crisp organic product.

• An early in the day bite is absolutely discretionary. On the off chance that you have a bigger breakfast, you may not feel hungry until noon. In any case, in case you're feeling somewhat ravenous and lunch is as yet a few hours away, a light early in the day bite will hold you over without including a great deal of calories.

• Lunch is frequently something you eat at work or school, so it's an extraordinary time to pack a sandwich or remains that you can warmth and warmth. Or on the other hand, on the off chance that you purchase your lunch, pick a solid clear soup or crisp veggie serving of mixed greens.

• A mid-evening tidbit is likewise discretionary. Keep it low in calories and eat only enough to shield you from inclination too hungry in light of the fact that supper is only a few hours away.

• Supper (aka dinner) is the point at which it's anything but difficult to over-eat, particularly on the chance that you haven't eaten much during the day, so watch your segment sizes. Rationally separate your plate into four quarters. One-quarter is for your meat or protein source, one-quarter is for a starch, and the last two-quarters are for green and beautiful vegetables or a green serving of mixed greens.

• A light unpredictable starch rich night bite may enable you to rest yet stay away from overwhelming, oily sustenance or nourishments high in refined sugars.

A Week of Healthy Meal Plans

Considering a couple of models may make the subject of dinner arranging simpler, so here's an entire week's value. You don't have to pursue the days all together; you can pick any feast plan, avoid one or rehash as you like.

The current week's feast plan was intended for an individual who needs around 2,100 to 2,200 calories for every day and doesn't have any dietary limitations. Your everyday calorie objective may fluctuate. Realize what it is underneath, and you can make changes to the arrangement to accommodate your particular needs.

Every day incorporates three suppers and three bites and has a solid equalization of starches, fats, and proteins. You'll likewise get a lot of fiber from entire grains, organic products, vegetables, and vegetables.

Each arrangement incorporates three dinners and three bites to keep you feeling fulfilled throughout the day. A few days even incorporate a glass of lager or wine. Don't hesitate to include more water, espresso or home-grown tea to quickly, yet remember that including cream or sugar additionally includes calories.

It's OK to swap out comparative menu things, yet remember cooking techniques. Supplanting a sirloin steak with flame broiled chicken is fine, yet supplanting it with pan fried steak isn't getting down to business in light of the breading changes the fat, carb and sodium tallies and the calories.

At long last, you can alter your caloric consumption by disposing of tidbits on the off chance that you need to get thinner or eating bigger bites in the event that you need to put on weight.

The very beginning

The present feast plan contains around 2,250 calories, with 55 percent of those calories originating from starches, 20 percent fat, and 25 percent from protein. It likewise has around 34 grams of fiber.

☐ Day One

Breakfast

•   One grapefruit

•   Two poached eggs (or fricasseed in a non-stick container)

•   Two cuts entire grain toast with one pat margarine each

•   One cup low-fat milk

•   One cup of dark espresso or home-grown tea

(Macronutrients: around 555 calories with 27 grams protein, 63 grams starches, and 23 grams fat)

Snacks

•   One banana

•   One cup plain yogurt with two tablespoons nectar

•   Glass of water

(Macronutrients: 360 calories, 14 grams protein, 78 grams sugars, 1-gram fat)

Lunch

• Chicken bosom (6-ounce partition), prepared or broiled (not breaded or browned)

• Enormous nursery plate of mixed greens with tomato and onion with one cup bread garnishes, bested with one tablespoon oil and vinegar (or serving of mixed greens dressing)

• Glass of water

(Macronutrients: 425 calories, 44 grams protein, 37 grams sugars, 9 grams fat)

Snacks

• One cup carrot cut

• Three tablespoon hummuses

• One-half bit of pita bread

• Glass of water or home-grown tea

(Macronutrients: 157 calories, 6 grams protein, 25 grams sugars, 5 grams fat)

Supper

• One cup steamed broccoli

- One cup of darker rice

- Halibut (four-ounce divide)

- Little garden plate of mixed greens with one cup spinach leaves, tomato, and onion beat with two tablespoons oil and vinegar or serving of mixed greens dressing

- One glass white wine (ordinary or dealcoholized)

- Shining water with lemon or lime cut

(646 calories, 42 grams protein, 77 grams starches, 8 grams fat)

Snacks

- One cup blueberry

- Two tablespoons whipped cream (the genuine stuff—whip your very own or purchase in a can)

- Glass of water

(Roughly 100 calories, 1-gram protein, 22 grams sugars, 2 grams fat)

☐ Day Two

In the event that you eat this entire menu, you get around 2,150 calories, with 51 percent of those calories originating from sugars, 21 percent from fat, and 28 percent from protein. The supper plan additionally has 30 grams of fiber.

Breakfast

• One entire wheat English biscuit with two tablespoons nutty spread

• One orange

• Huge glass (12 ounces) non-fat milk

• One cup of dark espresso or home-grown tea

(Macronutrients: roughly 521 calories with 27 grams protein, 69 grams sugars, and 18 grams fat)

Snacks

• Two oats treat with raisins

• Glass of water, hot tea or dark espresso

(Macronutrients: 130 calories, 2 grams protein, 21 grams starches, 1-gram fat)

Lunch

- A turkey sandwich (six ounces of turkey bosom meat, huge tomato cut, green lettuce and mustard on two cuts of entire wheat bread

- One cup low-sodium vegetable soup

- Glass of water

(Macronutrients: 437 calories, 59 grams protein, 37 grams starches, 6 grams fat)

Snacks

- One cup (around 30) grapes

- Glass of water or home-grown tea

(Macronutrients: 60 calories, 0.6 grams protein, 12 grams starches, 0 grams fat)

Supper

- Five-ounce sirloin steak

- One cup pureed potato

- One cup cooked spinach

- One cup green bean

- One glass brew (standard, light or non-liquor)

- Shining water with lemon or lime cut

(671 calories, 44 grams protein, 63 grams starches, 18 grams fat)

Snacks

- Two cuts entire wheat bread with two tablespoons jam (any assortment of natural product)

- One cup non-fat milk

- Glass of water

(Roughly 337 calories, 14 grams protein, 66 grams sugars, 3 grams fat)

☐ Day Three

The present dinner has around 2,260 calories, with 55 percent of those calories originating from sugars, 20 percent from fat, and 25 percent from protein. It likewise has 50 grams of fiber.

Breakfast

- One medium grain biscuit

- One serving turkey breakfast hotdog

- One orange

- One cup non-fat milk

- One mug dark espresso or home-grown tea

(Macronutrients: around 543 calories with 26 grams protein, 84 grams sugars, and 15 grams fat)

Snacks

- One crisp pear

- One cup of enhanced soy milk

- Glass of water, hot tea or dark espresso

(Macronutrients: 171 calories, 6 grams protein, 34 grams sugars, 2 grams fat)

Lunch

Low sodium chicken noodle soup with six saltine wafers

One medium apple

Water

(Macronutrients: 329 calories, 8 grams protein, 38 grams sugars, 17 grams fat)

Tidbit

One apple

One cut Swiss cheddar

Shimmering water with lemon or lime cut

(Macronutrients: 151 calories, 5 grams protein, 21 grams sugars, 6 grams fat)

Supper

8-ounce serving of turkey bosom meat

One cup heated bean

One cup cooked carrot

One cup cooked kale

One glass of wine

(784 calories, 84 grams protein, 76 grams sugars, 3 grams fat)

Tidbit

One cup of solidified yogurt

One cup crisp raspberry

(Around 285 calories, 7 grams protein, 52 grams sugars, 7 grams fat)

☐ Day Four

Before the part of the arrangement, expend around 2,230 calories, with 54 percent of those calories originating from sugars, 24 percent from fat, and 22 percent from protein. You'll additionally get around 27 grams of fiber.

Breakfast

One cup entire wheat piece with one cup non-fat milk and one teaspoon sugar

One banana

One cut entire grain toast with one tablespoon nutty spread

One cup of dark espresso or home-grown tea

(Macronutrients: around 557 calories with 18 grams protein, 102 grams sugars, and 12 grams fat)

Tidbit

One cup grape and one tangerine

Glass of water, hot tea or dark espresso

(Macronutrients: 106 calories, 1-gram protein, 27 grams sugars, 1-gram fat)

Lunch

Fish wrap with one wheat flour tortilla, one-half can water-pressed fish (depleted), one tablespoon mayonnaise, lettuce, and cut tomato

One cut avocado

One cup non-fat milk

(Macronutrients: 419 calories, 27 grams protein, 37 grams sugars, 19 grams fat)

Tidbit

One cup curd (1-percent fat)

One new pineapple cut

Four graham wafers

Shining water with lemon or lime cut

(Macronutrients: 323 calories, 29 grams protein, 38 grams starches, 5 grams fat)

Supper

One serving lasagna

Little garden plate of mixed greens with tomatoes and onions beat with one tablespoon serving of mixed greens dressing

One cup non-fat milk

(585 calories, 34 grams protein, 61 grams starches, 23 grams fat)

Bite

One apple

One cup non-fat milk

(Roughly 158 calories, 9 grams protein, 31 grams sugars, 1-gram fat)

☐ Day Five

This delightful feast plan incorporates three dinners and three bites and has roughly 2,250 calories, with 53 percent of those calories originating from starches, 25 percent from fat, and 21 percent from protein. What's more, heaps of fiber—more than 40 grams.

Breakfast

One-piece French toast with one tablespoon maple syrup

One mixed or poached egg

One serving turkey bacon

One cup squeezed orange

One mug dark espresso or natural tea

(Macronutrients: roughly 449 calories with 16 grams protein, 57 grams sugars, and 18 grams fat)

Bite

One cup cut carrots

One cup cauliflower piece

Two tablespoons farm dressing

Glass of water, hot tea or dark espresso

(Macronutrients: 223 calories, 4 grams protein, 18 grams sugars, 16 grams fat)

Lunch

Veggie burger on an entire grain bun

One cup northern (or other dry) beans

One cup non-fat milk

(Macronutrients: 542 calories, 38 grams protein, 85 grams sugars, 8 grams fat)

Tidbit

One apple

One pita with two tablespoons hummus

Shimmering water with lemon or lime cut

(Macronutrients: 202 calories, 5 grams protein, 41 grams sugars, 4 grams fat)

Supper

One trout filet

One cup green bean

One cup dark colored rice

One little garden serving of mixed greens with two tablespoons plate of mixed greens dressing

One glass of lager

Shimmering water with lemon or lime cut

(634 calories, 27 grams protein, 78 grams sugars, 13 grams fat)

Tidbit

One cup curd

One crisp peach

(Around 201 calories, 29 grams protein, 16 grams sugars, 2 grams fat)

☐ Day Six

The present suppers and tidbits have around 2,200 calories, with 55 percent of those calories originating from starches, 19 percent from fat, and 26 percent from protein. You'll additionally get around 31 grams fiber.

Breakfast

One cup corn drops with two teaspoons sugar and one cup non-fat milk

One banana

One hard-bubbled egg

One mug dark espresso or home-grown tea

(Macronutrients: around 401 calories with 18 grams protein, 72 grams sugars, and 6 grams fat)

Tidbit

One cup plain yogurt with one tablespoon nectar, one-half cup blueberries, and one tablespoon almonds

Glass of water, hot tea or dark espresso

(Macronutrients: 302 calories, 15 grams protein, 46 grams starches, 8 grams fat)

Lunch

One cup entire wheat pasta with one-half cup red pasta sauce

Medium nursery plate of mixed greens with tomatoes and onions and two tablespoons serving of mixed greens dressing

Glass of water

(Macronutrients: 413 calories, 11 grams protein, 67 grams starches, 12 grams fat)

Bite

One and one-half cup curds

One new peach

Glass of water

(Macronutrients: 303 calories, 43 grams protein, 23 grams starches, 4 grams fat)

Supper

Four and one-half ounce serving of pork midsection

Little garden plate of mixed greens with tomatoes and onions bested with two tablespoons oil and vinegar (or serving of mixed greens dressing)

One little prepared sweet potato

One cup asparagus

One glass wine (normal or dealcoholized)

Shining water with lemon or lime cut

(500 calories, 46 grams protein, 35 grams starches, 10 grams fat)

Bite

Five graham wafers

One cup non-fat milk

One cup strawberry

(Roughly 279 calories, 10 grams protein, 50 grams starches, 3 grams fat)

□ Day Seven

The present menu contains around 2,200 calories, with 54 percent of those calories originating from sugars, 22 percent from fat, and 24 percent from protein. There are additionally 46 grams fiber.

Breakfast

• One cup cooked cereal with one-half cup blueberries, one-half cup non-fat milk, and one tablespoon almond fragments

- Two cuts turkey bacon

- One cup non-fat milk to drink

- One mug dark espresso or home-grown tea

(Macronutrients: around 442 calories with 26 grams protein, 59 grams starches, and 14 grams fat)

Tidbit

One cup plain yogurt with one tablespoon nectar, one-half cup strawberries, and two tablespoons almond bits

Glass of water, hot tea or dark espresso

(Macronutrients: 343 calories, 17 grams protein, 41 grams sugars, 13 grams fat)

Lunch

Six-ounce heated chicken bosom

Enormous nursery serving of mixed greens with tomatoes and onions and two tablespoons plate of mixed greens dressing

One heated sweet potato

One entire wheat supper roll.

Glass of water

(Macronutrients: 498 calories, 47 grams protein, 63 grams sugars, 6 grams fat)

Tidbit

One cup crude broccoli floret

One cup crude cut carrot

Two tablespoons veggie plunge or serving of mixed greens dressing

One crisp peach

Glass of water

(Macronutrients: 112 calories, 3 grams protein, 25 grams sugars, 1-gram fat)

Supper

3-ounce serving of heated or barbecued salmon

One-half cup dark beans

One cup Swiss chard

One cup darker rice

One entire wheat supper moves with a pat of margarine

Shimmering water with lemon or lime cut

(671 calories, 38 grams protein, 91 grams sugars, 19 grams fat)

Tidbit

One Orange

(Around 62 calories, 1-gram protein, 15 grams sugars, 0 grams fat)

MINDFULNESS EATING

Regardless of whether you need to abstain from gorging and picking up those additional pounds, you have to control your glucose (for instance, in the event that you have diabetes), or you basically wish to devour just what your body requires, the Christmas season can make that objective testing.

Yet, careful eating may enable you to arrive at it.

Mindfulness alludes to the act of staying alert and at the time. Very regularly, our musings meander some place other than where we are at the time. Maybe we are engrossed with what happened an hour back, stressed over what may happen tomorrow, or worried over what we have to do one week from now. Care urges us to see these distractions, and after that to delicately take ourselves back to the now.

Care can help you completely appreciate a supper and the experience of eating — with control and restriction. A few examinations recommend that care-based practices help improve dietary patterns. For the individuals who pig out or eat for solace or out of pressure, careful eating may even guide with weight reduction.

Here are 10 hints for progressively careful eating. Not these tips may feel directly for you — attempt a couple and perceive how they work.

1. Reflect.

Before you start eating, pause for a minute to think about how you feel. Is it true that you are hurried? Pushed? Tragic? Exhausted? Hungry? What are your needs, and what are your needs? Separate between the two. After you have taken this minute to reflect, at that point you can pick on the off chance that you need to eat, what you need to eat, and how you need to eat.

2. Sit down.

Try not to eat in a hurry. Sit down. You're less inclined to value your sustenance when you are performing multiple tasks. It's likewise hard to monitor the amount you are eating when you nibble in a hurry.

3. Turn off the TV (and everything else with a screen).

Have you at any point looked down from your telephone or tablet or PC, just to ponder where all the nourishment went? These diversions make us less mindful of what and the amount we are eating.

4. Serve out your bits.

Oppose eating straight from the pack or the crate. In addition to the fact that it is simpler to indulge when you can't perceive the amount you've had; however, it is additionally harder to completely value your sustenance when it is avoided see.

5. Pick the little plate.

You may long for less on the chance that you see less. Littler plates will assist you with your bit control — a particularly decent technique for those everything you-can-eat buffets.

6. Give appreciation.

Before you begin to eat, respite and pause for a minute to recognize the work that went into giving your supper — be it because of the ranchers, the assembly line laborers, the creatures, mother Earth, the culinary specialists, or even your allies at the table.

7. Bite multiple times.

Attempt to get 30 berates of each chomp. (30 is a harsh guide, as it may be hard to get even 10 berates of a significant piece of oats!) Take time to appreciate the flavors and surfaces in your mouth before you swallow. This may likewise help forestall gorging by giving your gut time to send messages to the cerebrum to state you're full.

8. Put down your utensil.

Regularly, we are now setting up the following piece with our fork and blade while we are still on our past nibble. Take a stab at putting down your utensils after each nibble, and don't lift them back up until you have appreciated and gulped what you as of now have in your mouth.

9. Leave from the Clean Plate Club.

A significant number of us were raised to get done with everything on our plate and were not permitted to leave the table until we did. It's alright to drop your enrollment to the Clean Plate Club. Think about pressing the scraps to go, or simply leaving the last couple of nibbles. Despite the fact that no one gets a kick out of the chance to squander nourishment, overstuffing yourself won't help those out of luck. (This is additionally where Tip #5 proves to be useful.)

10. Quiet.

Take a stab at eating your dinners peacefully on occasion. At the point when it's peaceful, it is normal for the brain to meander; recognize these considerations, and after that check whether you can tenderly come back to your experience of eating. Be aware of the nourishment's consistency, flavor, tastes, and scents, and completely value the occasion. Obviously, supper time can be a significant time for sharing the day when the entire family accumulates, so having a whole dinner peacefully may be unreasonable or simply feel unbalanced. In any case, notwithstanding spending the initial five to 10 minutes peacefully can be reviving and established a thankful pace for the remainder of the dinner.

Conclusion

We need food to live, but we shouldn't live for food. We shouldn't depend on food as our main source of happiness and emotional stability. When that happens, our lives are out of balance and we aren't able to deal with our feelings on a deep, authentic level. That's the real reason why emotional eating can be a problem. There are other negative consequences, but when you depend on food for comfort, you're only soothing and not healing. Eventually, ignoring your feelings and not dealing with them in a healthy way makes life very challenging.

In this workbook, we went through what emotional eating is, its symptoms and consequences, and how to deal with it. There are four main emotions behind emotional eating - boredom, stress, anger, and depression - but for many people, their emotions are complicated and multifaceted. The exercises, practices, and journal prompts in this workbook still apply. It's up to you to listen to your feelings and identify what works best.

Deciding to tackle your emotional eating and pay more attention to yourself - both physical and mental - is a very bold and brave step. When working through this book and any other resources you find, always remember to be compassionate and patient with yourself. There will be times when you don't live up to your own expectations, but that's okay. Keep believing and keep pushing. Change is possible and you deserve to live your best life.